A DOSE OF MY OWN MEDICINE

A DOSE
OF MY OWN
MEDICINE

PAUL CAMPBELL

GROSVENOR
OTTAWA * SALEM Or
LONDON * MELBOURNE * WELLINGTON

First published 1992
GROSVENOR BOOKS CANADA
Suite 405, 251 Bank Street
Ottawa, Ontario K2P 1X3

GROSVENOR USA
3735 Cherry Avenue NE
Salem, Oregon 97303

GROSVENOR BOOKS
54 Lyford Road
London SW18 3JJ

21 Dorcas Street
South Melbourne
Victoria 3205, Australia

PO Box 1834, Wellington
New Zealand

Designed by Blair Cummock
Cover Design by Cameron Johnson

Canadian Cataloguing in Publication Data
Campbell, Paul, 1912—
    A dose of my own medicine

ISBN 0–9695852–0–9

    1. Campbell, Paul, 1912–   . 2. Physicians—
Canada—Biography.   3. Moral Re-Armament (Organization)
4. Christian Life
I. Title.
R464.C35A3 1992   610′,92   C92–090119–0

British Library Cataloguing–in–publication Data:
A catalogue record of this book is available
from the British Library

Phototypeset in Sabon by Intype, London
Printed and bound in Canada by Tri-Graphic Printing (Ottawa) Ltd.

To the Native People of Canada and every Canadian from coast to coast.

ACKNOWLEDGEMENTS

I want to thank Irene Massey, for her tireless typing and retyping of my first manuscript, and her ever-cheerful and willing spirit. My gratitude especially goes to Virginia Wigan, who has done a masterful job of researching, ordering and editing the manuscript. Without her expertise this book would not have seen the light of day. I am grateful too for the skill and insights of many friends, including Elizabeth Locke.

And last but not least I value the frank and affectionate criticism of my wife and my two daughters.

PSC

CONTENTS

INTRODUCTION

IN THE CANADIAN WEST, where the Rocky Mountains meet the prairies, a Native Canadian woman sat by the bedside of her sick son. There was no way she could have a qualified doctor attend the boy, or bring him to the hospital. The sum involved was out of the question.

The white man's regulations said that she, an 'Indian' on a Reserve, was entitled only to a 'medical chest' which the Indian Agent, a political appointee, had in his control. It was little better than a First Aid kit, and could not save her boy. A second son was also stricken, and died without seeing a doctor.

A devout woman, she and her husband had prayed day and night for their children to be saved, but they died just the same. Belief in God was shattered and anger against the white man welled up in their hearts.

In the early years of this century a young Englishwoman went to Canada to be married to a Scots Baptist pastor. The daughter of a city merchant, she was ill-prepared for the rigours of prairie life, but adjusted fast. She raised her children to have faith in God, and with her husband created a wonderful home.

Tragedy struck when their little girl contracted influenza and died, at the age of five. In those pre-antibiotic times the doctor was powerless to save her. The Alberta winter freezes the ground to iron, so the child's body had to lie out on the porch of her home till the earth was soft enough for her grave to be dug.

In the same years a Swiss family emigrated to Canada. The teenage daughter and her new husband created a farm on virgin land in the Gaspé Peninsula of Québec. They built a log cabin from trees they cleared at the end of a dirt track,

1

deep in the forest and four-and-a-half miles from the nearest village. The stony ground did not easily lend itself to cultivation, unlike the fertile prairie lands of the English-speaking settlers in the west.

In the unforgiving heart of a January snowstorm the woman went into labour. Her husband rushed to get the doctor – arriving back just as the baby had been delivered by his sister-in-law. Fearing for its life in the freezing weather, the doctor advised the young couple to wrap the child well and lay it on the open door of the oven . . . the simple method which saved many a new-born babe in those parts. In spite of great hardships the family grew up in a happy home, true poineers of French-speaking Canada.

I was born into this vast diversity that is Canada. It was my little sister whose body lay through the winter days and nights on the porch of the house. I was only seven when she died, but I had already decided that I was going to be a doctor.

Chapter One
A FORD MODEL 'T'

MY FATHER, Don Campbell, who became a Baptist pastor with various parishes in Western Canada, was one of 12 children born to the blacksmith on the island of Canna in the Inner Hebrides in Scotland. In those days Canna had a population of 300, for whom the main source of income was the pasture land on which cattle and sheep grazed.

At the turn of the century there was not enough work on the island for all the young people. My Dad found a job in London, and went to Spurgeon's College to study for the Ministry.

He wanted to pioneer the Gospel in an area where, if he did not go, there would be no messenger. He was invited to Alberta, Canada – to the prairie town called Vegreville, where I was born. The house where we lived, remodelled, still stands.

My mother came from Leeds, Yorkshire, taught school in the Channel Islands, and followed her fiancé to Canada, where they were married in 1911 in Winnipeg, in a double wedding with her sister. I was born in 1912, on the very night the Titanic went down. My sister Edith was born in 1914.

Our mother was a great personality – a gifted musician both at the piano and with her lovely singing voice. She could speak like an angel – full of fun and really dedicated in her support of my Dad's work. She taught Sunday school – taking the classes which no one else could control. She gave me a very great heritage, with her strength of purpose and faith. For that I am eternally grateful.

She was a little taller than Dad, and very elegant. He was short and robust and strong – in the springtime he would hit practice 'fly' balls with a baseball bat for the local kids to catch.

Dad was very easy to talk to. He used to do the handyman

jobs around the house, and I would help him. And my parents were very happy together. They were very different in character – where Mother was artistic and musical, and very practical about things like the family accounts, Dad was more rough and ready. He loved to work on the farms of his neighbours and friends, especially at harvest-time.

In those days, the minister's house was the centre of a lot of communal activity. People would come in through the kitchen door, and get a cup of tea and sit and chat. One man came in and sat down, and Mother offered him a bowl of fruit. She was quite taken aback when he ate the lot.

Mother gave piano lessons to some of the local children, as a way of augmenting the family finances. In our home on Saturday nights some of the neighbouring farmers would come in and sing together while Mother played the piano – it was more than just a sing-song, those men could really sing well. We had many an evening like that.

At Christmas time we always had a house full of people, especially on Christmas Eve, with Dad the life and soul of the party. We children would go skating or sleighing – and then come in for food and music.

As pastor, my father would receive many invitations for Christmas dinner, which he always accepted. One year we had 14 Christmas dinners – turkey, plum pudding, Christmas cake – in 14 different homes on 14 different days. It certainly was a Christmas for a boy to remember.

In winter in Alberta the lakes froze over so hard that the people were able to go out onto the lake and make a hole in the ice to fish through. I remember those nights, when the snow crackles underfoot and glistens like a carpet of tiny diamonds under the clear sky with its sparkle and light.

It was in the 'Spanish influenza' epidemic of 1919 that Edith – aged five – was stricken.

My parents took turns in the night watching over her. The doctor came, but could do nothing. I shared a bed with my Dad. One morning as I wakened he said in a choked voice, 'Edith left us last night.' As she died she had said, 'I love Jesus.' Her next breath was her last.

My sister's death was in winter. Two or three times a day, my father or mother would put oil on the face and body of their dead child as she lay on the porch at home, awaiting

4

burial. Imagine the heart-ache they must have endured during those days.

I have missed Edith. She was five, I was seven, when her life ended. We were good companions and enjoyed much fun together. It was lonely without her.

Mother spent all her days during that epidemic nursing neighbouring families. All members of a household could be ill at the same time, with no one well enough to prepare food. The virulence of the illness was such that strong farmers coming by wagon to buy groceries in the morning could be dead that evening. We all wore masks, to try and gain some protection from the infection.

Edith was buried in the Vegreville cemetery, where today beside her rest my father and mother. Dad loved children, and perhaps he saw in every small child after that the daughter he had lost. What I do know is that from then on my parents' care for people of all ages was deepened and widened.

One of Dad's parishioners, a bachelor at the time, was Ben Hawkins – a farmer from England. He had a very good tenor voice, and was one of those who often came to our home to sing around the piano while Mother played. Ben was at Edith's funeral. I saw this big rugged farmer grasp Dad's hand as they stood beside the coffin. That moment is indelibly etched in my mind.

Mother and Dad would drive by horse and sleigh in the winter. On one occasion while they were out travelling and night was beginning to fall, Dad said, 'I think we will go and stay at that house over there.'

'Do you know them?' enquired Mother.

'No,' replied Dad.

They knocked at the door but no one was home. They went in, made a meal, slept for the night and left the next morning, having written a note to the owner saying who they were and what had happened. That was the way people operated in the West in those days. But Mother was never very sure about it.

In those early years Dad went everywhere in a carriage drawn by a team of horses. Mother often went with him. Once on the way home from visiting a parishioner in the countryside, he was pursued by a prairie fire carried forward by the wind. These fires could go at an incredible speed when there was a wind, feeding on the dry grass and copses of bush. Dad escaped due to the speed of his team, but he did have a scare.

His whole objective in life was to pass on his faith to his friends. He was single-minded in that. He went to work with the farmers because he loved it, not because he was preaching or pushing. Yet his sermons were forthright, and did not pull any punches on sin or salvation.

He was a real fighter and had a rare spirit. He completely trusted God and loved him – he spent a lot of his time on his knees and with his Bible. What men think counted little with him if it didn't measure up to what he had learned of the Almighty and his way of life. He's a type we could do with a lot more of in this old world.

It was not until we visited the island of Canna many years later that I fully understood Dad – his habit, for instance, of shouting across the street to greet people he knew in Edmonton, or even people he didn't know. It embarrassed my mother, because it just wasn't 'done'. But in Canna, a small community where everyone knew everyone else, you naturally greeted people as you went around, and you greeted them loudly.

Some months after Edith's death Dad, Mother and I moved to Lavoy, not far from Vegreville, where I went to school. It was a town of about 300 – 400 people, where the kids from all the surrounding farms came to school. Dad was the minister.

Lewis Bricker, the Jewish proprietor of the local General Store, was a good friend of Dad's. They would have long talks as to who crucified Christ – the Jews or the Romans. In times of economic depression Lewis would accept no cash from the farmers – he extended credit, and usually they would pay up when times were better. In those days everyone had to be good neighbours to survive.

Once I went into the store and pocketed some candy. When I got home I got a good strapping – and I dare say I was made to return such of the candy as I had not already eaten. I am still in touch with the son of that store-owner. Another day I came home from school with some tennis balls which did not belong to me. The loss was noticed, and I was given a few licks with my father's old razor strap.

Mother volunteered to teach the Chinese man who brought the vegetables to our door to speak English. He would come to our home two or three times a week. One Sunday he decided to visit Dad's church. Being a bit shy, he thought the most inconspicuous approach would be to come through what seemed to be the back door of the church – only to find himself standing in the pulpit. Dad took him down to a front seat and made him welcome. I don't remember the poor chap coming back, however.

After breakfast every morning we used, as a family, to read the Bible and then get down on our knees and pray. One fine morning as we were all kneeling, I looked up irreverently and longingly at the summer's day outside the window. Suddenly I caught sight of our neighbours setting off on a picnic – so I quietly tiptoed out to join them. As my parents had their eyes closed at the time they did not know where I had gone.

When I was eight or nine I used to work with the man who ran the Grain Elevator – tidying up his desk, running errands for him and so on. Then one day I made a small platform to fit on my little handcart, so that I could fetch groceries from the train when it arrived and deliver them to the General Store. As I was paid for that service, I guess it was my first job.

I had a dog called Jeff, and I was sometimes called Mutt, after two cartoon characters of the day. We were inseparable. But one day he got into the shed where we kept the horses' feed, ate the poison put down to kill the rats, and died. It was terrible and I wept and wept. A neighbour, realising what I was feeling, kindly gave me a small black water-spaniel.

At Lavoy the school was just across the way from our home. One evening when I was eight my parents called me to the kitchen window where, with mixed feelings, I watched my school burn down. It was later discovered that the furnace, kept going all night in the winter, had started the blaze. From then on our schooling took place in local churches and homes, wherever there was space for a classroom.

7

I used to go out shooting partridge. Once I had a near miss when I stumbled with the loaded gun in my hand. It went off and the bullet nicked my shoe.

We children would sometimes pour water down the gopher holes and when the little creatures came rushing out we'd try to whack them over the head.

I still remember the coyotes howling on the long winters' nights. Sometimes, I think because it was supposed to be healthy, I was tucked up on the porch to sleep, and I remember waking up with my eyelids frozen together.

My mother looked after the chickens. I guess I must have had chores to do – I do remember chopping wood. Also clearing the pathways of snow in the winter. I remember the summer hay-rides – the church social picnics and bonfires.

I think I was named after St Paul – maybe my parents hoped that I would end up somewhere in the mission field.

But my decision to be a physician was made at the age of six. The only man in Vegreville with a car, a Ford Model 'T', was the local doctor. Any time he visited our home, I would be found sitting in the car as he was about to leave. I used to love dispensing bottles of coloured water as 'medicine'.

Then Dad was called to the Okanagan Valley, a lovely part of British Columbia with low hills – a fruit-growing area, producing the famous BC Delicious apples. We lived in Armstrong, famous for its celery, most of which was shipped to Vancouver and Chicago.

In High School at Armstrong, with medicine in mind, I took Greek and Latin (surgery has many words rooted in Greek, while medical words are rooted in Latin). Once I was asked to recite 'amo, amas, amat . . .' while the teacher threw pieces of chalk at me. He said it was to test my concentration.

I was a moderately good athlete, playing baseball – I was pitcher and short stop, soccer and track running on school teams in the summer, and ice-hockey, basketball and badminton in the winter.

Once, catching a ball in a baseball game, I received the ball on the end of a finger, which is crooked to this day. I broke my nose playing ice-hockey – the puck hit it or a hockey stick, I suppose. That is still noticeable also.

I liked to study, and relished the challenge of exams. When

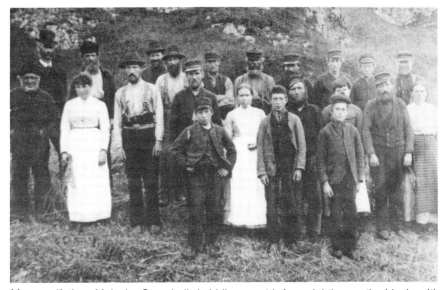

My grandfather, Malcolm Campbell, (middle row, 4th from right), was the blacksmith on the island of Canna.

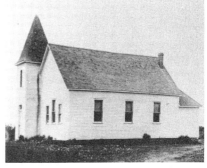

Lavoy church. 'My father wanted to pioneer the Gospel in an area where, if he did not go, there would be no messenger.'

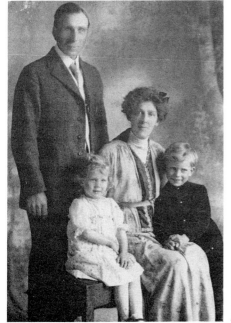

My parents, Don and Annie Campbell, my sister Edith, aged 4, and myself aged 6.

the family moved to Vancouver, where Dad was called to a church in 1928, I entered the University of British Columbia to read zoology and chemistry, and such courses best suited to a medical career: biology, physics and so on. The most interesting course to me was that of making slides from animal tissue for staining and microscopic study.

Fortunately I could include some Latin, philosophy and English Literature in my studies. When later I became fully involved in the medical curriculum there was no time for these subjects. I was also a member of the University debating team. We travelled to Winnipeg for a debate, which we did not win, on the resolution that the civilization of the west is a greater menace to the world than that of Russia. We also debated by radio with the University of Alberta in Edmonton.

In my final year at the University of BC I applied for but did not receive a Rhodes Scholarship. But I had good academic grades, and was also able to continue my athletics, competing at inter-University level at the half-mile and 440-yard distances.

I graduated with a BA degree in the class of 1932.

My first job in Vancouver with my degree was the elevated position of delivery boy on a bicycle for a 'drug store'. The store did a roaring trade in rubbing alcohol, which I would deliver – often to elderly ladies. From time to time I pondered whether they actually rubbed it on aching parts of their anatomy, or drank the stuff. At any rate, for this service I received the princely sum of $1 a day. I was lucky to have a job at all, in those days of the depression, and $1 bought a great deal more than it does today.

In spite of the fact that I often spoke at young people's church rallies and was President of the Inter-Varsity Christian Union, I had become disillusioned by church activity – particularly by the unhealed animosities between and within churches. I was on the way to becoming something of an agnostic. The great debate amongst the Baptists, between those with a more liberal theology and the 'fundamentalists', divided my Dad's church in Vancouver and resulted in his resignation. There was no financial provision in those days for pastors without a congregation, so his was a difficult decision. However, a short time later he was offered a pastorate in Alberta.

In that year, 1932, I went to a service in the First Baptist Church in Vancouver, to hear people known as the Oxford Group. Their acknowledged leader, whom I saw but did not meet at that time, was Frank Buchman – a Lutheran pastor from Pennsylvania. The idea that stayed in my mind after that service was 'God has a plan – you have a part'. That meeting made an impression on me – something to do with the size of Buchman's aim, his method of going about it, and his sincerity. These people were lively, with an infectious high-spiritedness, and they were interested in affecting the state of the nations, beginning with individuals.

One day the pastor of that same First Baptist Church in Vancouver asked to see me, and enquired if I would be interested in accepting a student pastorate at a small church in Olds, Alberta. It was only two hours by train from Edmonton and the medical school at the University of Alberta, and so I jumped at the chance – I needed any money I could get to pay for my tuition. Around the same time Dad was called back to Alberta, to be pastor in a farming community, something he hugely enjoyed – working in the fields when he could. He and Mother were there during all my medical school days, 60 miles away from the University of Alberta.

I still have the letter my Mother wrote to me for my 21st birthday.

April 13th, 1933, Vancouver
My dear Son,

Many happy returns of your birthday. May this new Cycle of your life begin and continue with the happiness you have had in the past 21 years and its success also. You would do well to remember Longfellow's lines:

'Let me then be up and doing
With a heart for any fate,
Still achieving, still pursuing,
Learn to Labour and To wait.'

The hardest lesson in life is to learn to wait especially for the young mind, but it is a valuable lesson when learned.

'Let no man despise thy youth, and be thou an example of the believers, in word, in conversation, in love, in spirit, in faith, in purity. Neglect not the gift that is in thee. Take heed to thyself and unto the doctrine, continue in them, for in doing this, thou shalt both save thyself and them that hear thee.' I Timothy 4.

God has signally blessed you, my son, and I believe He has a great task for you to do in these days which are becoming more and more difficult. Never let go of God. He is.

The prayers of your Father and Mother follow you day and night.

With a great love, Your Mother.

There was a good Badminton Club in the town, which I joined and enjoyed. The manager of the bank was a friend and competitor at the Badminton Club, and it was he who introduced me to the game which became my favourite sport – golf. My Dad and I would sometimes go out and hit a few balls together on the golf-course.

I had good congregations, though my talks in the church were more to do with situations in the Province, country and history than with theology – for which of course I had no formal training.

My weekend schedule was a punishing one. First I had to get out to Olds, where there was a Sunday morning service, followed by a 20-mile trip to give an afternoon talk in the countryside, then an evening service on return to Olds. Then I took a 3 am train to Edmonton, to be on time for my first lecture at 8 am on Monday morning. After a week of lectures and laboratory work I would return to Olds on the Friday evening to meet with a group of young people.

The organist and her husband, the postmaster, were good friends. He would take me hunting, and tried to teach me to shoot grouse on the wing. They have been life-long friends.

I got to know the farmers who made up my 'flock', as well as the drug store proprietor, the hardware merchant, the bank manager and his family, the Roman Catholic priest, the Methodist pastor, and the principal of the school who asked me to coach the school basketball team.

After my second year in medical school it was just not possible to carry the pastorate and my studies as well, so I resigned the church work. However this meant I needed to earn enough money in the summer months to pay my university fees. The Provincial Minister of Agriculture offered me a job to teach at Olds Agricultural College during the summer. I learned far more of economics, Canadian history, English Literature than my pupils did – because I had to swat it up in order to be able to teach them. I was given board and room. And my salary made it possible for my medical studies to continue.

While at medical school in Edmonton I made many friends, not only in the school but also in the city.

On Saturday afternoons, with lectures and laboratory work at rest, many of the 31 in our class would meet at someone's home for beer, ping-pong, and discussion. Once I tried to grow a moustache, but it turned out red, and my class put me on the floor of the anatomy lab and shaved half of it off. So that was the end of that.

I was one of five in my medical class selected to intern at our University Hospital in Edmonton. We lived in a dormitory on the top floor of the hospital, subject to call at any hour of the day or night. We received room and board but no salary. The urological service always seemed to have patients who during the night would require catheterization to relieve bladder pressure. For many weeks I was on call. It was arduous, after a full day in the wards and attending clinics and lectures.

One night I was called to deliver a young woman, about 19 years old, who had attempted an abortion. She died as she expelled the dead child from her womb. I thought of her family and their pain. It left an unforgettable mark on my life.

We were increasingly exposed to clinical work during our final two years. Our obstetrics and gynaecology professor – a Dr Conn – got more book work out of us than any of the others. But after attending seven deliveries between the hours of 2 and 4 am, I decided that on the whole obstetrics was not for me.

The professor of neurosurgery was so precise in diagnosis that his speciality appealed to me. But after seeing some of his post-operative cases, when the success-rate in the field of neurology in the late '30s was not very high, I was disillusioned by the results.

Our professor of orthopaedics was giving us a clinic one

day when someone went by the door whistling. The professor rushed out to stop the offender, muttering as he re-entered the room, 'A hospital is no place to be cheerful'!

The head of dermatology, a Dr Menagh, whose department dealt with venereal disease, had an extremely penetrating voice. I can still hear him, behind closed doors, explaining to a patient in tones which echoed up and down the corridor, 'Confidentially, you have syphilis!'

Dr Menagh suggested to me that I should write my own text book of medicine, studying typical cases in depth – with laboratory and X-ray findings – write them up with the preliminary diagnosis, and the autopsy findings if the patient did not survive. I carried out this suggestion, which taught me a lot.

Once while I assisted at an operation the surgeon inadvertently nicked the renal artery. A stream of blood like a geyser shot into the air. The haemorrhage was speedily dealt with, and the patient seemed no worse for the incident.

It was around this time that the first antibiotics, sulfa drugs, came into use – you could spot those on sulfa by the blue tinge to their skin.

We had a dull professor of pharmacology. His lectures really were sleep-inducing. He was also anaesthetist at the local hospital, where a fellow-student, by the name of Welwood, was taken for an appendectomy. When he saw the professor approaching to anaesthetise him, Welwood said, 'Don't bother with the anaesthetic – just read me one of your lectures.'

As part of our training we had two weeks internship in a mental hospital. One day I was making rounds in this hospital. I passed two patients in the corridor, and heard one of them remark, 'I do like that fellow – he's so like one of us!'

However, the professor who caught my imagination was the professor of medicine. He arrived at the hospital in a chauffeured car, with a small dog beside him. He had an entertaining way of presenting his lecture material, and often illustrated it with actual patients. This I felt was my field – who knows what influence the chauffeured car had? It may have been a memory from my childhood attraction to a Ford Model 'T'. In any event, my ambition developed to be a professor of clinical medicine at some prestigious university.

Chapter Two

UNDER THE MICROSCOPE

IN THE SUMMER of 1934 I was scheduled to help run a boys' camp with a man I had never met. He lived in Edmonton, and invited me to spend a weekend in his home so we could get to know one another. Certain features of his character recalled to my mind the Baptist Church meeting I had attended in Vancouver two years earlier. Whereas I was concentrating on my career, he was concerned not primarily with himself, but with the country – its unity, policy and people. Till then I thought such concerns had nothing to do with medicine or with me – that was the job for the politicians.

He was also interested in how I was going to use my medical training. This coincided happily with my own chief preoccupation. I started asking questions, to see if this interested quality of his was inherited or acquired. He interrupted me. 'You know,' he said, 'you and I are exactly alike.'

'We're very different,' I replied. 'That's why I am asking these questions.'

'No', he said. 'People are the same inside whatever the colour of their skin, their beliefs, their backgrounds or their history. Human nature is the same everywhere on earth. We can love and hate. We can be greedy or we can sacrifice. We can be dirty or clean. I think I am finding the way of allowing the positive elements in my nature to dominate more readily.'

I was interested, for I knew only too well I had failed to match my living with my ideals, and with those of my parents.

I asked how he had discovered this ability. He told me that he had looked at his motives, his habits, and relationships, his aims, under the microscope of absolute moral standards – the standards Christ outlined in his Sermon on the Mount: honesty, purity, unselfishness and love. 'That's no good to me,' I told him, 'because I do not accept the absolute in the moral field.'

'But the world does,' he replied. 'If you try to pay less for next term's tuition than is required, you won't get in.'

'But supposing I was to try this idea of yours, where would I begin?' I demanded.

'Oh, that's simple,' he answered at once. 'You came into this life with two ears and one mouth. You need to listen twice as much as you talk – to the Almighty and to your neighbours.'

'Listen, to the Almighty?' I repeated. 'Do you mean hearing voices? In medical practice we have special hospitals for those people.'

'You may hear a voice,' he replied, unruffled, 'but more likely you will get an idea. It may be one you've had before. This time, do something about it.'

I returned to my room at the University residence, and – convinced more by the man's personality than by his philosophy – I decided to make the experiment. I took four large pieces of paper. This idea of looking at my life under the microscope of absolute moral standards filled me with apprehension. It might turn out to be a lengthy and depressing analysis.

Strangely, I had but one thought. It was that I had two books in my room which I had picked up in the University bookshop and taken home without paying for. Medical books are expensive, and I had but little money.

The next day I met my new friend again. He asked me how the experiment had turned out.

'It doesn't work for me,' I answered. 'The only thought I had was about two medical books I had taken without paying for. There are several things in my life which I consider worse than stealing. So, if the experiment really works, why did I not have ideas about beginning where I feel I need it most? You see,' I added, getting into my stride, 'basically I am an honest man – it's the thing I am proud of.'

'You may think you are honest,' he said, 'but you sound like a thief to me.' His honesty jolted me into reality. I returned the books to the proprietor saying, 'These belong to you not to me.'

'Thank you,' he responded. 'I lose a lot of books from here in a term. You are the first one ever to bring any back. Why did you do it?'

'I'm not sure,' I told him, 'but I am trying an experiment – to be absolutely honest.'

'Good God!' he exclaimed. 'Sit down and tell me all about it.'

He got his books back, and I made a friend. More importantly, it was the beginning of a realisation that there was a dimension to life that I had been missing. It was definite, clear, almost too practical, and it produced results. What more could a medical man want? It made me feel as if I had life by the tail.

Shortly after I returned the books to the bookshop, I was walking down the street near a classmate's home. He had a charming young wife and two children. My friend, Doug Cameron, stopped me in the street. 'Campbell, you're different. What's happened to you?'

'I've just had a haircut,' I said.

'No, what I'm talking about is the look in your eyes.'

I started to tell him of my experience with the stolen books.

'Wait,' he said, 'come into the house so that Agnes can hear.'

They both began to listen to what God had to say to them. One day she came out with startling honesty. She was so fed up with his selfish behaviour that she had been considering taking the children and rejoining her parents in the East. Doug was thoroughly shaken. It was the beginning of a better communication in their life together. Agnes stayed.

Their honesty awakened in me a resolve never to take people for granted. In our beer sessions in their home, it had never occurred to me that our host and hostess had reached such a precarious stage in their relationship. I was too wrapped up in what I was doing to notice. When Doug died, a few years later, the family was completely united.

My next thought of consequence was that I should tell my parents the difference between the way I behaved at home and at University. At home I neither smoke nor drank, for instance. At University I did both. Then there were the girl friends, the nurses, the dances.

It was not easy for me to be honest. I knew the facts would hurt them. Since my sister's death they had centred their hopes and pride on me. Their response to my honesty moved me deeply, and bound us even more closely together.

Dad asked me, 'What is it that you have found that you didn't receive here at home or in our church?'

I answered, 'Not a blooming thing, except that these people have shown me the way to make it all practical.'

My parents gave me a gold ring to mark the deeper degree of trust and solidarity in our relationship.

I was still at medical school when I first suggested to Dad that we should have a time of listening together. After some minutes of quiet I said to him, 'Dad, what came to you?'

He replied, 'Not a darn thing!'

I said I didn't think it was possible for someone to sit on their bottom for 10 minutes without a single thought in their heads.

'Oh' he said, 'I had lots of thoughts!' The first was a verse from the Bible, 'Those that ascend the hill of the Lord need clean hands'.

I asked, 'Dad, where do you need cleaning up?'

He got quite agitated at that suggestion. When he calmed down he said, 'I think I should go and apologise to a man down the street who belongs to a different denomination, because we have not been friends for 14 years.' And he did.

I was plagued with a very short temper. I could get livid at what I perceived to be injustice. Never once did I have any thought about how to deal with my temper. It just faded away – and has not returned. As I put right what I could put right, the Almighty must have put right what I could not. These simple experiments began to rekindle my faith in the Almighty. When I listened and obeyed, the results were evidence of a Power at work in me beyond my own resources. I knew myself well enough to know that any thoughts that could pass the test of those absolute moral standards could not have come from me.

The time of listening to the deepest thing in my heart and mind – which I believe to come from God – became for me a vital part of starting each day, and has remained so for the rest of my life. It is not solely a matter of putting right what has been wrong, essential as that is. It is the only way I know to chart my life's course and my day's work, and above all to strengthen my relationship with Christ. However inadequately I do it, it is a life-line.

In the summer and winter of 1936 several young Canadians who had been intrigued by the Oxford Group would meet at the local YMCA for basketball and a swim, ending with a time in which we would share our thinking, the things we had been up to and so forth.

In June 1936, some of us went to an Oxford Group meeting in Stockbridge, Massachusetts. A meeting of several hundreds was suddenly startled by a crisp, clear voice interrupting the proceedings from the rear. Frank Buchman had just entered. 'Open the windows. Open the windows, It's stuffy in here.' He came over as both definite and authoritative.

A tall man in his late fifties, Buchman possessed an urgency, a clarity and conviction on what was needed, that was totally foreign to the mentality of the Canadian West at that time. He hit me like a cold shower.

Frank Buchman was born into a Pennsylvania Dutch family. He studied at a theological seminary, and then chose social work in one of Philadelphia's toughest areas, where the Lutheran church asked him to create a hospice for destitute boys. They were hard to handle, and they were hungry. Money was short, and Buchman came up against the six members of the finance committee in charge of the hospice, who ordered that further economies should be made – on food. In vain Buchman sought to have more money released, and finally he resigned in bitter frustration. His health began to fail, and on medical advice he took a cruise around the Aegean. His resentment against the six men on the committee continued to eat away at him, and his life-work seemed in ruins.

He travelled to Britain, hoping to meet a certain well-known preacher who might be able to help him. He never found the preacher, but one Sunday in Keswick, in the Lake District, by chance he went into a small chapel where a middle-aged woman was preaching to a congregation of 17 people.

'She unravelled the Cross of Christ for me that day', said Buchman. 'The doctrine I had known as a boy came to life through her. I saw the great gulf separating me from the sorrowing Christ, and I knew it was because I was nursing ill-will. I thought of the six committee men. I hated them with a cruel hatred. I asked God to change me, and he told me to put things right with them. I left the chapel with a consciousness of having the complete answer for all my sins. I walked out of that place a different man.'

He went to his room and wrote a letter to each of the six men on the committee, asking their forgiveness for having nursed ill-will against them. While their actions were wrong, he realised he himself was the seventh wrong man because of his resentment. He reported that as he posted the letters it was as if a heavy load was removed from his back. Suddenly he was free.

His effective work with individual men and women began that same afternoon, when he told a young man, the son of the house where he was staying, what he had experienced. The young man, who was regarded as something of a 'problem', in turn opened his heart to Buchman, and the afternoon ended with the young man committing his life to God.

It was in the early 1920s that Buchman first met and made friends for life with students at Oxford – continuing his simple, direct, personal work with everyone he met. While the numbers of people whose lives were affected by coming into contact with Buchman were relatively small, the very nature of their radical thinking and approach to life made them a by-word in the University. It was not long before 'The Oxford Group' came into being – the name attached to Buchman and his colleagues by a newspaper-man while they were on a visit to South Africa.

One day at Stockbridge I decided to introduce myself to Buchman and I went up to him as he was leaving a conference session. I held out my hand and said, 'My name is Campbell. I am a University student from Western Canada. I have wanted to meet you.'

'Hello,' he replied, shook my hand, and walked on.

That was all. I don't know what I expected. Perhaps the conciliatory bonhomie which I was accustomed to. But this was firm, brusque, businesslike, and one thing was clear – he was a man with a mission. I could participate if I wished, but there would be no cajoling. It would be my decision, based only on my own conviction.

It seemed irrefutable logic that if I wanted to change things, the best place to start was with myself. I had already begun to learn that. And the notion of applying absolute standards to my society suggested the most radical social, political and economic revolution I could conceive of – something in which everyone was needed. Personal faith, important as I knew it to be, was not enough. When I looked at my own small start, taking back stolen books, I realised that, were it multiplied around the town and around the nation, a world revolution would be in the making. What could be more important?

Two months later, in August, Buchman spoke to America by radio from London. With Hitler, Mussolini and Stalin in everybody's minds, and some believing that a dictator might be good for the democracies, he gave his conviction – 'Many have been waiting for a great leader to emerge. The Oxford Group believes that it must be done not through one person, but through groups of people who have learned to work together under the guidance of God.'

Our Edmonton youth meetings culminated in a camp in 1937 on the grounds of Regina College in Saskatchewan. Sleeping tents were provided by the Royal Canadian Mounted Police and a cooking tent and utensils by the Army. Young men came from all over Canada, from Vancouver to the Maritimes.

While at that camp some of us had in mind to make a movie illustrating our convictions. Cece Broadhurst from the University in Winnipeg wrote tunes and words which he would sing with his guitar – he was to play the role of a cowboy; another student from Ottawa, Ted Devlin, took the role of a student, while I was cast in the part of a truck driver. The theme song of the film was written by Ted Watt, author and one-time journalist with the *Edmonton Journal.* The film was named *Youth Marches On.*

Also with us in Regina was a gifted musician, a Scot named George Fraser. He told us he felt we ought to go to England, to a large youth gathering at Oxford that summer, an Oxford Group house-party. While in England we planned to complete our film in studios near London, which had facilities Canada could not provide.

25 of us decided to go. To raise our fares we sold possessions and insurance policies; some business and labour men made contributions which enabled the 25 to go by train to Montreal. Someone gave us an old refrigerator for the trip, and at the train stations we passed through friends would come with gifts of food. My own travelling fund was

the gift of a railway station master, a man named Stevenson. He was convinced of the value of our plans, having known the Oxford Group for some time.

We went steerage across the Atlantic from Montréal to Plymouth, which was quite an experience. I had got together various medical supplies, as the doctor to the group, and I handed out cotton balls for people to put in their ears, because the ship's whistle was so loud. One man was afraid he was going to die – he had never been on a boat. Then just one day out at sea and he was afraid he wasn't going to die. It certainly was a rough ride.

While crossing the Atlantic we received a cable from a Canadian friend, anxious that we should not be an embarrassment to the British – 'Disembark quietly and proceed to Oxford'. There's no question that my time in England with the young force had a lot to do with my conviction about being ready to join Buchman. We all lived in tents in a large field – I recall vividly some of the characters we met. They were a lot of fun.

It was the general impression I got of the group in Oxford that attracted me, the way they cared for one another, and everybody around them. It was their quality of life, the friendship and the camaraderie amongst them that was so infectious. They had such fellowship, and they were ready to serve one another. The only time I had experienced anything like it was in my own home.

They were men and women who had decided to give their whole lives to serve God, some of them at considerable cost to their personal careers or financial status. None of them were paid, but were supported by others who believed in the work they were doing. Some of them had been with Buchman for many years, travelling far and wide with him, and undertaking the same personal, nation-affecting work. It seemed to me to be a great privilege to be part of the same happy band.

It was also mind-stretching, as we had people from different parts of Europe, and even some from South Africa there. And of course it was a great experience for me to come to Britain for the first time, the place where my parents had their roots.

The Oxford Assembly was where I saw Buchman again,

but at a distance, sitting with the Marquis of Salisbury. At the first session we Canadians were invited to speak.

Buchman was never prominent in that conference. He always had other people doing the speaking and taking the lead.

But he also used the assembly to train a force of people. His method was simple, straightforward, clear. I found myself noting down some of his words: 'Some of you hinder things by being too cautious'. 'You can be like a traffic light – green with envy, yellow with softness, red with resentment.'

He would ask searching questions, 'Can you expect national leaders seriously to consider your work as an answer to world needs?' 'What would happen to industry, education, the country, if everyone worked at your pace?' 'To what national problem are you demonstrating an answer?' 'What do you really expect to happen in the world as a result of what you do?'

Again, he would emphasise – 'You need a strategy. The answer of the Holy Spirit for any given situation at any given moment to any given person. A divided mind comes from a disordered life – the devil will do anything to water us down.'

He had advice on studying the New Testament, which he considered was the revolutionary handbook of all time.

We had about a month in England that time, and returned to Canada with some of the Englishmen. We travelled across Canada and saw politicians and others en route. We wanted to tell them of our experiences and our new-found vision for our country. We had to sit outside the office of the President of the Canadian Pacific Railroad all day, in Montréal, waiting for an interview, and we took turns in having lunch. At 4 o'clock in the afternoon he said, 'I'll see you now.'

We had a reception given by the Government of Canada in Ottawa, and some of us went through the line twice so that we could have further conversations with the dignitaries.

Our film of *Youth Marches On* was shown all over Canada by the 20th Century Fox chain, as well as in Britain and across India and Australia. Its European première was in Geneva at the League of Nations. Incidentally, the film is now in the archives of the Canadian Film Board, as the first Canadian musical on film.

Our time in England laid the foundations of a faith that

has stood the tests of war and the relaxations of peace. Several of the group lost their lives on the battle fronts of Europe.

Chapter Three
ONE MORE GOOD DOCTOR?

WHILE WE YOUNG Canadians were still in England, I cabled the head of the University Hospital in Edmonton to ask if my leave could be extended. I received a curt reply that my post at the University Hospital had been given to another.

However, at the conference in Oxford I had had the privilege of meeting Dr Frank Sladen, chief of the Medical Staff of the Henry Ford Hospital in Detroit. This prestigious institution was a hospital certified by the American Medical Association for the training of specialists in all fields.

On returning to Canada, I wrote to Dr Sladen to see if there might be an opening for me on his staff. The immediate reply I received was that, if I could be there by June 1, there was an internship available. So I went, forfeiting the graduation exercises in Edmonton, and began my work in internal medicine in June 1938.

Dr Frank Sladen had been at the John Hopkins Medical School and houseman to the famous Canadian physician, Sir William Osler. Sladen had been asked by Henry Ford to create a staff for the hospital Ford was building. Naturally, he brought his colleagues from John Hopkins.

Henry Ford was not impressed by the way the head of a patient's bed was raised – the old deck-chair technique. He returned a few days later with a wheel which, when fixed at the end of the bed, could be turned to raise or lower the patient. Today, of course, in some hospitals you just press a button and the head of the bed moves to suit the patient's convenience. In the Nurses' Home which Ford built there was another pioneering new feature – every nurse had her own room and bathroom.

My appointment to the Henry Ford Hospital turned out to be a marvellous four years. The training consisted of spending several months in each of the various medical specialities – psychiatry, cardiology, gastro-enterology, dermatology, general medicine, haematology, the pulmonary system, general circulatory system, glandular disorders. We had 600 patients in the wards. In addition, up to 1000 patients a day came to see us in the out-patient departments.

The patient who did the most for me as I made the rounds was the one who said to me, 'Campbell, I think you are a good doctor. You know what you're doing. But couldn't you give more of yourself to the patients?'

When I first began the practice of listening I had a thought that transformed my medical work and my relationship with everybody – 'give as much interest to the patient as you have been giving to the disease'. After all, it is not illogical to think that the purpose of medical science is people. There is a sick society as well as sick people to attend to. It is all-too easy for a doctor to climb his career ladder by making use of a person's illness, rather than primarily being concerned with the welfare of his patient.

I owe a great deal to Frank Sladen, who had great faith in my medical future. He took me under his wing, grooming me for a top career. He took me with his family on holiday trips to New Hampshire. On a Saturday afternoon he and I often went to Ann Arbor for the University of Michigan football games. Not infrequently I was invited for dinner in his home. He encouraged me to attend medical conferences in different parts of the country where I could meet leaders of the medical profession in America. He and Mrs Sladen could not have been better friends, and indeed treated me like a son.

I actually proposed marriage to his daughter, but she turned me down, to my chagrin. She may well have wondered, not without reason, how much was my devotion to her and how much was devotion to my career.

My mother, on the other hand, had hopes of my marrying a local Edmonton girl. She wrote to me about it one day, during the war years, while I was in Detroit.

August 8th, 1940, Lavoy

My dear Paul,

Catherine has a new Ford V8 1940 and drives beautifully, and Paul, she is the loveliest girl I think I ever met – she has everything – looks, charm, refinement, cleverness, spirituality, and anything else you can think of that goes to make up the sweetest piece of femininity one could desire. Why in the world you don't secure her for yourself is beyond my powers to imagine. Both she and her mother certainly think a lot of you, if you need any encouragement in the matter.

Yours joyously, Mother.

In 1940 the head of a well-known clinic in Calgary came to Detroit, to see me at the Ford Hospital. He took me out to dinner at a down-town hotel and invited me to join his clinic as an internist. It was an attractive proposition – with my roots in Alberta, and Calgary is in glorious country, within easy reach of the Rocky Mountains.

As I left the hotel dining room, whom should I meet but my physician-in-chief, Frank Sladen. He offered me a lift home. 'What did that man want?' he enquired.

'He invited me to join his clinic in Calgary.'

'Well' said Sladen calmly, 'I think your career might be better served by staying with us!'

So there I was, with a decision to make. What I actually did was to write to Frank Buchman, a man whose perceptions and assessments I had come to respect. Though I did not know him personally, I wrote asking his opinion on which choice I should make regarding my career.

He replied, saying that if I listened for God's plan I would be shown what was the right course. The trouble was, I felt I had been listening, and had been rewarded only with uncertainty.

But two days later Buchman sent me a second letter, suggesting that perhaps there might be a third option in addition to the two I had before me. The effect was to remove the pressure of having to decide. I could wait – an alternative which had never crossed my mind.

I was grateful also in those years for the support and encouragement I always received from my parents. Times were hard for them, financially, and my Mother worked wonders in balancing the family budget as she did. I was glad to be able to help them out from time to time, as my own resources permitted.

27

March 8th, 1940, Lavoy
My dear Son,

Your very interesting letter came yesterday. I knew when you were home that you were not so spiritually minded as you were the previous visit, and the thing that impressed me very much was the effect your state of mind had upon your father and I, for all the time you were home we did not have our morning reading and prayer more than twice if that many. Such a thing never happened before in all our lives or since. It certainly is true that no man lives to himself and how little we know how we are unconsciously influencing others . . . I am so grateful to God that you have come to see the truth, not Self but Christ. Gal. 3:20; Gal. 4:26; Phill. 4:13. God bless you and guide you.

Today we have a real March day snow and blow. I broke my glasses the other day. I should really have my eyes tested again – but until the car is paid everything else has to wait. This month my boarder goes home for Easter for 10 days, that means $10 short in the house-keeping. If I should ask for a loan until end of July of $10 at the end of this month, should I meet with a favourable reply? We owe only $200 now (for the car) and are paying $50 a month so it will all be paid for by end of June.

Our boarder is to be married in July so we shall not have him next term. I shall be glad. I have felt very sick for two days, but am more like myself tonight. The Vitamins you are sending have not arrived. It is a month since I had any. They must be held up in Customs. We are very delighted at your appointment because it means you have done the right thing all along. I suppose it will mean more salary and you can begin to save for your future home.

Now son, Never lose sight of Jesus Christ.

Cheerily and joyfully – Mother.

March 18th, 1940, Lavoy
My dear Paul

Thank you very much for the enclosure in your last letter . . . . Last Sunday Dad got into a snowdrift and of

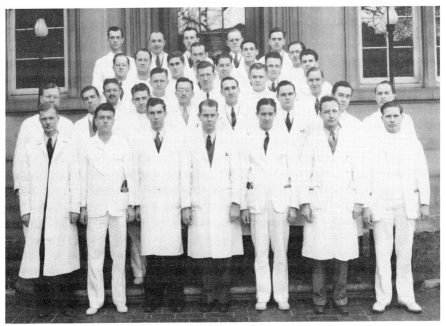

'My appointment to the Henry Ford Hospital turned out to be a marvellous four years.'

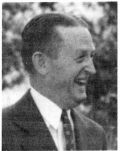

'I owe a great deal to my chief-of-staff, Dr. Frank Sladen.'

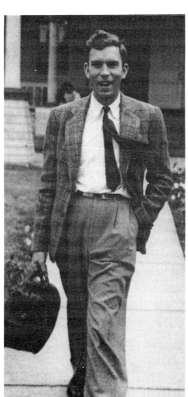

'My ambition was to be a professor of clinical medicine at some prestigious university.'

course as usual he stripped his gears and has to have a complete new transmitter. He got home at 10 pm so I had to be preacher for the evening service. I enjoyed it and I think the listeners did too, at least they said so. I got the Vitamins you sent me on Wednesday, had to pay 58 cents duty.

Much love – Mother.

April 4th, 1940, Lavoy
My dear Paul,

. . . Thank you from Dad and I for the $10. I got $11, less the exchange, for your cheque. One could make money just now – $110 Canadian for $100 American. American money is worth 10% more here . . . Isn't it grand to serve God whole-heartedly. Some people have just enough religion to make them miserable. A complete surrender brings joy and peace.

Oceans of love, Joyously yours – Mother.

November 13th, 1940, Lavoy
Our dear Boy,

We hope you are not over-working, because a doctor cannot afford to neglect his own health. It was too bad your patient didn't respond to all your care and attention.

It will soon be Xmas. I was thinking that if you and I could get Dad an overcoat it would be so helpful – his old coat is done. I think I could get one from Vancouver for $15, and I have had some back music lessons' money which I meant to spend on a new dress but I should have greater joy in putting it into an overcoat for Dad. If you think you could help, just send a message to say 'OK Xmas is near' and I will write and see what they have. You can put my Xmas present into Dad's for he does need a coat – make it a gift for both . . .

Oceans of love, Joyously yours, Mother.

While I was working at the Henry Ford Hospital, I followed Buchman's activities, and those of the Oxford Group, with intense interest. The world broadcasts he made, the mass-meetings before the war in Denmark, Holland, Sweden, Switzerland, Birmingham, and Oxford; his publication of a pictorial magazine which went in one-and-a-half million copies in eight languages to heads of state on every continent.

The building of a new world was for him the logical consequence of one person finding a new moral structure to their living and a new source of direction, for such a change immediately affected the person's family and the society in which he lived and worked. And he was a realist. He could see that the experience and purpose which had gripped him was a decision facing each new generation – and would be to the end of time.

In 1938 he launched his programme under the title of Moral Re-Armament.

It is hard to see how one man without official position of any kind could have done more to prepare the world for the crisis that was upon it. During the war Buchman worked intensively in America. In 1940 he was saying 'Our task is to enlist everyone in America's war – the war for industrial co-operation and national unity. Nothing less than this must be our aim.' A musical revue with the theme of 'sound homes, teamwork in industry, unity in the nation' was taken to every major city in the country. Round table conferences were held with leaders of management and labour, meetings, newspaper articles, radio broadcasts and person-to-person work was conducted across the nation.

In 1941 I was invited to an assembly in Cleveland, Ohio, where Buchman was bringing together some 200 of his team of people. At the suggestion of government and Defence Councils, his men and women had been at work in the shipyards of the East coast and in the aircraft factories of the West coast, with the aim of raising morale in the homes and workplaces of the people who lived there.

The Cleveland assembly was called to review the situation in the country and to see together what further action to take. I began to sense that I could be part of a world-wide force of people committed to seeking God's will for the national life.

Buchman was convinced, after the evidence of two world wars and a depression, that there was not enough wisdom in mankind to extricate us from our follies by political, economic and social programmes alone. He knew first-hand that there was added intelligence available when people sought it by paying the price morally in their own lives. From that conviction he never wavered – it was the aim that dominated all his relationships.

He was certainly the most interesting, the most single-minded person I had ever met. I had rarely known a man possessed of so much energy. He was always up early in the morning and often retired late at night. He would move in and out of a room so quietly you did not miss him till he was gone. He had the faculty of being able to give his best to the person he was with at the moment with insight and sensitivity. He could sense what I was feeling even before I was aware of it myself.

At this weekend in Cleveland I had a brief conversation with Buchman. I asked him what would be the outcome of the war. He said, 'Because of her industrial strength America will likely be on the side that dictates the terms of peace. But unless America changes, she will lose the peace.'

Then he looked at me. 'Young man,' he said, 'what this country needs is not just one more good doctor. It needs an answer to selfish materialism, for without it we may win the war but we will certainly lose the peace.'

My mind was jolted with the impact of a new idea.

In fact, the first medical encounter I had with Buchman was at the Dearborn Inn, Michigan. His team were in Detroit to give a performance of the musical revue *You Can Defend America* in a downtown theatre. I was full of training from the Ford Hospital. My chief-of-staff in medicine had definite ideas on the diet best suited for maintaining and sustaining health – a breakfast largely of fruit, a lunch which emphasized vegetables, and a meat or fish course at dinner. I had observed Buchman's choices of food, and noted they did not really accord with my chief-of-staff's recommendations. Here was a man brought up in the Pennsylvanian traditions of serving the best food available, in the best possible quantities. Presumptuous of me as it was, I went up to Buchman while he was having his breakfast and expounded my ideas of diet.

'That's what I do!' he interjected. 'Good food and good Christianity go hand in hand!'

I retreated, with the wind rather taken out of my sails.

In 1942, while still on the Ford Hospital staff, I attended a conference in Richmond, Virginia. I went to thank Buchman, and to say goodbye on the Sunday evening. I had to be back at work in Detroit on the Monday morning, and I also had a research project lined up at the University of Michigan, and lectures at the Wayne County Medical School in Detroit.

Buchman asked, 'Have you had guidance from God to go?'

I replied I didn't need God to tell me what to do – I had obligations to meet. He suggested we listen to God together.

After a few moments he enquired, 'What thoughts did you get?'

So I restated my position, 'My thought is to go.'

'That's strange,' he said, 'mine was stay, stay, stay. Let's listen some more.' This time I came up with my reasons and arguments why I had to leave. Again he repeated, 'Stay, stay, stay. We're divided on that one, aren't we? Should we pray together?'

So we did.

As we were quiet, deep down I knew I was experiencing an undeniable sense of calling to join Buchman in his work. I thought of my effort, as a loyal son of the Empire, to enlist in the Canadian forces on the day war was declared in Britain. I had not been accepted, probably because they were looking for more experienced physicians at that stage. Then I thought, 'The Americans will likely soon be calling me up to serve in their Armed Forces. Whether I have obligations in Detroit or not, I will be leaving the hospital – so why not make the break now?'

That decision was the toughest I ever had to make. To break with Dr Sladen's encouragement and advice, together with the disappointment I knew I would cause him by turning my back on a promising medical career, made it an extremely difficult decision for me.

My parents were disappointed also. Sladen had outlined to them how he saw my career in medicine developing – and at the time they did not fully understand why I made the decision to give it up.

Sladen himself didn't say anything to me when he heard my decision, but a little later I had a telegram from him saying I had been appointed to the National Research Council, and would I accept? He may have been trying to get me back. I think he understood my decision, but was also disappointed.

When making that decision, the deepest conviction in me

– stronger for once than my ambitions – was that it was the right course for me to take. I have never regretted making that choice.

There was no training in nine years of University life for such a task. But I was completely convinced by what Buchman was doing, both its importance and its urgency, for the future of the nations.

Some 25 years later I visited the Hospital in Detroit. Frank Sladen was now an honorary consultant in medicine. I sat with him and Mrs Sladen in the main lobby, and we had a time of quiet together.

I will never forget what he said to me, 'We've come full circle, haven't we?' I owe the Sladens a great deal, for their life-long friendship, and for their encouragement in those early years of my medical career.

In the next immediate months in 1942 I saw more of the remarkable character of Frank Buchman. No action was ever planned and initiated without a sensitive search for God's direction. With him, it was such a natural procedure, and he moved with such alacrity and speed. He was totally unpredictable. For me, as with the others who worked with him, there was no salary attached. I worked with him on the basis that there was a job to be done, and I felt an inner compulsion to join him in it. And from that day to this I have found my decision to live by faith and prayer for my needs has been honoured by the Almighty, and also by my friends. I have had a life-time friendship with a man with whom I trained at the Henry Ford Hospital. He began sending me a cheque for $20 every month when I gave up my position at the hospital – a gift I received regularly until he died.

In my time with Buchman, one of the chief characteristics was merriment. Like Old King Cole, he was a merry soul. He had a mischievous twinkle in his eyes – and the laughter of those with him was one mark of the comradeship he developed. It was the sheer joy of people who were free of wanting anything for themselves. And he had unbounded vision and faith. 'Campbell is a fine fellow, worthy of much improvement!' was one of his trick phrases.

On my first call-up I was given a year to continue my work with Buchman. At the second call-up I was rejected on an

X-ray finding. By this time I was fully engaged in Buchman's Moral Re-Armament work which had been described by the Secretary of the Navy as equal in importance with material re-armament.

In August 1942 I attended an MRA conference on Mackinac Island, Michigan. I looked out of the window one morning at breakfast to see Henry Harkins walking with his family by the lake-shore. Henry was a promising young doctor brought in to the Henry Ford Hospital from Chicago, and the hope was that one day he would take over the Department of Surgery. He and I had become friends through our mutual addiction to golf. But he had not been satisfied with the arrangements for his research work at the Hospital and became very critical of the staff who had built up the various specialities. One day Henry was called in to be told that he had created such ill-will among the staff that perhaps his career would be better served somewhere else. In the event he became an associate surgeon at the John Hopkins Medical School, where his first work was with the pioneer of infant cardiac surgery.

I rushed out from the dining-room at Mackinac to greet Henry and his family, and we arranged a golf game. During the game he offered to show me some new medical text books he had with him, so I returned with him to his hotel.

There I found that it was not so much the books he wanted to talk about, as the trouble he had had at the Ford Hospital and more lately at the John Hopkins. He asked if I could help him. He told me he believed that he could make a contribution to the science of medicine, but his bad relationships kept frustrating his best intentions.

I said I did not think I could help him, but I believed I could tell him how to get help. 'If we were to listen quietly to the deepest thing in our hearts, we could well be shown what to do,' I offered.

He said he would like to try. He had three thoughts:

1. To see his parents in Chicago who had not yet accepted his wife as part of the family. He went to visit them every year, but was more divided each time he left over the question of his parents' feeling of superiority to Jean, his wife. It arose because Henry was a doctor, and his wife was 'only a nurse'.

2. To write letters of apology to those members of staff of the Ford Hospital whom he had criticised.

3. To invite to a meal in his home the colleague with whom he was currently having difficulty at the John Hopkins.

Two years later I spent a night with Henry and his wife. He greeted me with, 'I wish you could have come a bit earlier – before my parents left. They have been staying with us, and we have had a wonderful visit.' He told me that his relationships with the staff were now so good that he had been asked to head up the surgical department of a new medical school in Seattle, where ultimately he co-authored a book on surgery which became a standard text in American medical schools.

The following year I received a letter from him, while he was Managing Editor of the Bulletin of the John Hopkins Hospital. He wrote:

'I can report distinct progress. I am not slipping back into the old ways nearly as much as I anticipated might be possible . . .

'In fact, I can see now that my whole daily program has been a mess and very inefficient: up too late, hurry to work, no time for planning, arrive late, rush around, get home late, be so exhausted (mainly mentally) that I would relax into a period of evening hours wasted reading newspapers and magazines. Much of this has been changed, much remains to do . . . there are endless possibilities for better work.

'Jean has at least a dozen times said that we have never gotten along so well as during the past six weeks.

' . . . There's one man, chairman of a committee that I am on, who had disagreed with most everything I said and with whom I didn't get on well. I met him a couple of days after my return with especial care, due to having prayed about this encounter, and sought direction from the Almighty on how to handle it. We now get along very well. The decision of the committee is now to be reversed to what I'm sure is right – so all is turning out well.

'Distinct progress has been made with my mother, at least I am being much more open with her and write regularly, rather than sporadically as in the past.

' . . . I hope to report more progress soon.'

Chapter Four
BUCHMAN'S PHYSICIAN

SIX MONTHS AFTER leaving the Henry Ford Hospital I was in San Francisco with a few others, preparing for the visit of a larger group. Buchman had sent me there to work with people concerned with industry, especially the men and women of the world of labour and the trade unions. I believe he felt I had something to learn from them which my medical degree had not taught me.

Suddenly a phone-call came which profoundly changed the course of my life. It was from Dr Irene Gates in Saratoga Springs, NY informing me that Frank Buchman had been taken seriously ill and would I come?

I arrived in Saratoga to find him in a coma. At 10.30 am on Saturday, November 21st, 1942 he had been walking along the corridor to the elevator when the man following him, his secretary, Morris Martin, saw him walking somewhat sideways. In the elevator he sagged, and was put in a chair when he got out of the elevator – otherwise he would have fallen to his right. He was returned to his room.

On my arrival that evening I was taken immediately to Buchman's bedside. He was critically ill, cyanotic, pulse rapid and completely irregular. There were râles in his lungs – the sound of moisture one hears when a stethoscope is placed over the lungs of a person in heart failure. The left side of his face was paralysed and his right arm and leg were motionless.

The next day, Sunday, at 3 pm he had a mild convulsion, and on Monday we secured an oxygen tent and suction apparatus to clear his throat. On the Tuesday he again had a slight convulsion, with marked cyanosis, was semi-comatose and by late evening was again in acute heart failure. With his speech slurred by his partial facial paralysis he said, 'I feel death close. I have seen the outstretched arms and they are wonderful. Have the funeral in Allentown (his home town) on Sunday or Monday.' Those of us with him prayed the Lord's Prayer. This episode was followed by a period of restfulness and contentment and was the beginning of a distinct gain physically. On November 25th I noted his lungs were clearer and he was gaining in strength.

From then on we could see signs of a return of the energy which had always been a feature of his life.

In the first few weeks Buchman needed 24 hour nursing. We brought in a trained nurse for the night duty. She was metallic and unsympathetic, more interested in the money than in her patient. The second morning, after the nurse had left, Buchman – with his impeded speech – murmured to me, 'Either she goes, or I do'.

She went. For when Buchman was conscious he was in complete touch with his environment.

Several times in those days we felt he was dying. On one occasion he called his closest companions around his bed. He asked for his wallet to be opened, and indicated whatever was in it was to be shared among us. It was all he had.

Before he had taken ill Buchman had been working with people in Washington on an important matter. Of all the hundreds of men who worked with him he put it up to the Government to keep some 30 of his most thoroughly-trained men free of military service, in order to continue and expand their work for the country. People made uncomfortable by Buchman's uncompromising message in Britain and America seized on this request as a means of insinuating that the men of the Oxford Group were involved in draft-dodging, pacifism and possibly subversion. The headlines broke across the front pages of the press shortly after Buchman rallied from the precarious state of his condition. He looked at the paper, smiled and said, 'We have a good team!', turned on his side and went to sleep.

The specialist, Dr Carl Comstock, asked me if Buchman was anxious. I certainly was, and said I thought Buchman might well be. Buchman's retort was, 'You don't understand how I feel!' He was annoyed by my remark, for it was not true. He had great peace of heart.

Once he complained of an upset stomach. I diagnosed

and efficiently prescribed. 'You don't know anything about stomachs, do you?' he rejoined.

As a matter of fact, I had worked with the gastro-enterology department at the Henry Ford Hospital for some months, and had a fair training in the subject. But I knew I could not, as far as Buchman was concerned, any longer rely on my special knowledge to prove my worth.

A bit later he remarked, 'You know, Paul, I don't think we are going to call you a doctor any longer.'

For him there was only one source of security, and it was not in a man's ability, position or training.

He would not tolerate, when he sensed it, any reliance on himself as a person, as a substitute for trust in the Almighty. Any time he sensed that I was depending on him for judgement or direction, I would find myself swiftly in the doghouse − instead of being appreciated, I could see I was a considerable annoyance.

During those days I found Buchman increasingly difficult to work with. Nothing I did met with approval. I began to be restless with a desire for a more personally-satisfying use of my life and profession. For if I was not to be considered a doctor, I had no reason for being with him. I realized that being seen as a doctor gave me a certain position, and a function without which I would be lost, that I was relying on some status or achievement for my life's meaning and purpose.

When he had improved enough we went with him to Washington, and the night we arrived there from Saratoga was, for me, the breaking point. I spoke with my friends. I had come to the end of the road. To Buchman I felt I was more of a burden than a help, and the best thing I could do was to clear out. Finally one of my friends, an officer on leave from the Infantry, asked me, 'What do you want for yourself?' I wanted to pull my weight, where I was needed, and in a way that was worthwhile. I wanted a modicum of appreciation and credit.

'Of course,' said my friend, 'you will be like that wherever you are.' I saw the truth of it, and decided to stay. In my spirit I knew I should.

The next morning, as usual, I was the first one in Buchman's room. No one had seen him since my decision, so he could not have known of it, but he was different. His whole attitude had changed. I was made to feel a welcome colleague, and so it remained.

He had a rich sense of humour and was incessantly pulling the legs of his friends. He called me 'Alpaca', referring I think to my Alberta heritage.

Shortly after I made my decision to stay with Buchman, he announced that he wanted to visit Miami to see three of his men graduate from officers' training school. In his condition it was not an easy trip. Going through Alabama by train he asked me what I preferred for breakfast – coffee or tea? I said 'tea', so we ordered tea. It was tepid, made from water off the boil, and quite undrinkable. Buchman left me to discover this, and then remarked, 'Now you have learned – when in the Southern States, always order coffee!'

His company was bracing because he was honest about what he was thinking, and never hesitated to express it. He was a very good friend. You felt you could be honest with him. Something he used to say was, 'You cannot live on yesterday's breakfast. Some people share the truth, but not what they believe or how they live.'

'A fellow who has guts enough to come and share his weaknesses – it shows that somehow or other he trusts you enough to tell you all the things in his life he does not like. It's a tremendous thing. I would do anything for a fellow like that. He can have my shirt or anything I have any day. That's the sort of people I would like you all to be . . . that I could come and tell you all about myself, and you would say you understand.' He wasn't judgemental – once when I told him of a moral slip his comment was, 'I'm so glad you told me.' He was quick to forgive and move on. He said to a group of us, 'Often God tells me I have been a fool, in no uncertain terms . . . .' (long pause) ' . . . often.'

He loved going for drives in the countryside, and would see birds on the trees which had escaped some of our younger eyes. He enjoyed people who were absolutely real, not pretending to be better than they were – like Rachel Jackson, his cook, who when he didn't eat enough would come and tell him off, after all her work in preparing the meal.

Before he had his stroke he was one of the most energetic people I had ever met – up at the crack of dawn till late at night, and he moved like quicksilver. That's one reason why I felt his stroke may have saved his life, because he had an irregular heart anyway and I am sure that if he hadn't been slowed down by his stroke he would have died much earlier from heart failure.

He was invigorating, never dull. He was fun to be with. He wanted others to enjoy the best on offer.

He liked music and he loved the stage and screen. He took a small party to a first performance of *Oklahoma* in a New York theatre. His aside about the heroine who sang 'I'm just a girl who cain't say "no"'!' was, 'I think we could help her!'

I enjoyed looking after him, bringing breakfast, helping him with all the details of daily life. He was always eager for world news. I would read him the morning newspaper – particularly the obituary column. And he was eager to get all his mail which Morris Martin would read to him every morning.

Buchman was interested in the individual – that was what concerned him. He always wanted to know how things had gone; when you had visited someone, he wanted an account of your conversation and how the person responded. However, he expected you to do it freshly. Once, when asking about an interview the previous day, he said to me, 'What did you tell that man – the same old thing?' There was a certain uniformity to life with Buchman. As he once put it, 'When I go on vacation it is a change of location, not a change of vocation.'

When a friend remarked how tired he had become during a conference, Buchman replied, 'I don't understand that. I live exactly the same way in a conference as I do when not in a conference.' It was quite true. Circumstances might differ, but because of his preoccupation with the human condition, his routine did not change.

In his last years he was often awake every two or three hours during the night, and would call me in. It was disconcerting to be wakened from the depths of sleep, to be asked on entering his room, 'And what have you been thinking about?'

Once, when some of us were fuming at a malicious innuendo launched by a British MP, Buchman said, 'Now let's pray for him. He needs help.'

41

He did admit that the first time he was publicly criticised it was like a knife-thrust. But later, he said, he found criticism bracing – 'it sets you up for the day'.

It wasn't that he believed he was always right, but he had a hatred of the lie. He felt that a deliberate smear was like poison-gas to the people who heard it.

Buchman did not drink or smoke. As a young man, growing up in his parents' small hotel, he had had every opportunity to drink, but as his work with people developed in effectiveness, he believed he could not be used to help the drinker if he himself was a sipper. On the other hand, once I was with him as house guests of a Swiss cigar manufacturer who said, 'I see none of your people smoke. Should I stop making cigars?'

Buchman answered, 'On the contrary, you should be making the best cigars in Switzerland.'

He did not change his principles – but he was always conscious of the particular person he was talking to at the time.

Another reason why he didn't drink or smoke was that he was frugal. His only personal expenses were things like getting his hair cut. Yet he was very lavish in hospitality and in seeing that the needs of those around him were met.

He knew from experience that where God guides he provides, and He knew that the Almighty provided not only the finance but the ideas and people when needed. This has proven to be true countless times in my own experience.

He never took anyone for granted, no matter how long they had been with him, or how effective they had been. When things were wrong he said so.

He once asked to see a young businessman who was working with him, and in the clearest and most forceful language upbraided him for buying more expensive than necessary boat tickets for some 50 people. When my friend could get a word in, he said, 'But Frank, you've got the wrong man. I had nothing to do with the tickets!'

'Well,' said Buchman with conviction, 'it's the way you would have bought them, if you had!'

He once remarked to his friends, 'If I had not been willing to risk my relationship with each of you – 24 hours a day –

we would not have a force of people committed to remaking the world.'

But indeed there was such a group of people, when he died in 1961, which I believe was used by God to bring healing and renewed purpose to individuals and to nations – to France, Germany, the Nordic North, Japan and the Philippines, Africa, and many places in between. For a fuller account of Buchman's life I recommend the biography written by Garth Lean of Oxford, *Frank Buchman – A Life* (published by Constable & Co, London, 1985).

In 1943 Mother joined me at an MRA conference on Mackinac Island, Michigan. Her curiosity had finally got the upper hand. For, although grateful for what had happened to me, she had her suspicions concerning MRA.

A lady who got to know my mother at the conference came up to me one day and asked me, 'Have you ever been really honest with your mother?' 'Certainly,' I replied.

'Well then,' she persisted, 'if you have, why does she still think you are such a wonderful fellow?'

I saw her point. I took Mother for a walk. I told her I wanted her to be rid of a false image she had of her son, and I began to tell her some of the things I had been up to during my time at the Henry Ford Hospital, associations with secretaries and nurses, and so on. I was deeply ashamed, and she was deeply hurt. She stopped me. 'I don't want to hear any more,' she said, and left me standing.

She did not come to lunch nor to tea that day, nor dinner.

'Of all the mistakes I've made,' I thought to myself, 'trying to be honest with Mother is the worst.'

But that same evening she knocked on my door. As I opened she began, 'I've come to apologise.'

'I'm the one apologising today,' I responded.

'No,' she explained, 'your father and I wanted to have a model Christian home so that you would have an example to follow. But we had our jealousies and particularly our differences of opinion concerning your upbringing and future. Now I see if we couldn't be honest with you when we were wrong, why should we expect you to be honest with us when you were wrong?'

That insight transformed her attitudes. Our honesty then

was the foundation for a rich relationship, the like of which we had never had before.

On her way home across the Great Lakes by boat she saw a nun on the deck. She had an inborn suspicion of Catholics and other denominations, but she decided to approach the nun. Mother wrote me with considerable surprise, 'We had a good chat. And you know, she holds Christian principles!'

That winter she sent me a wire for New Year: 'Joyous New Year greetings. Love to Dr Frank, Irene (Dr Gates), all the family. Much love. May all your dreams come true. God bless you. Mother.'

I was never to see her again for she died in January 1944 of a brain haemorrhage caused by high blood pressure. I was in New York when I had the telephone call. I was thunderstruck at the news. In fact, it was such a shock I could not continue the phone conversation. I set off immediately by plane to Lethbridge, Alberta, where Dr Hugh Arnold, a medical classmate, met me and took me to his home for the night.

The next morning, by train, I reached my father in Medicine Hat. Dad gave me Mother's wedding ring – which my wife now wears. We then travelled by train to Vegreville, where Mother was buried beside little Edith, beneath western pines looking over an unbroken stretch of western prairie as far as the eye can see.

Her funeral service had deep joy and power. Friends came many miles and filled the church to capacity. Neighbours and life-long friends were the pall-bearers, and the school was closed for the day in her honour. We had a bouquet of lily-of-the-valley and roses for her.

At the burial service Dad's last words to her were 'See you in the morning, Mother.' His faith shone through. I experienced a strange mixture of pain and joy – the pain of losing her and the sheer thankfulness for all she gave during the years.

Pain, given to Jesus Christ, can open our hearts in a fresh way. It is no problem – for when we share it, it is the bridge over which we enter each other's lives, the highroad into another person's heart. If we do not share it we let our friends go hungry.

Dad went to live with his old friend, Ben Hawkins, on his farm for a time after Mother's death. I did not like leaving him. Her death was like an amputation for him. They had been together for 34 years. But he insisted that I should rejoin Buchman.

When Mother came to Mackinac in 1943 it was the first time she really began to understand to what I had committed my life.

Some months after her death Dad also came to Mackinac for a visit. He met many of my friends, including Buchman and Bunny Austin, on leave from the American Air Force. Bunny is the British tennis star who, with his actress wife Phyllis Konstam, was giving all his time to Buchman's work. The story went round the assembly that Dad's handshake was so strong that he needed a doctor going round after him setting the bones of the hands he had shaken!

In 1944 *The Forgotten Factor*, an industrial play by Alan Thornhill, an Oxford don, was performed in the National Theatre in Washington, DC. The play tells a story of change in the manager of a factory and his family, and in the militant head of the Union and his family, and the consequent solution to their intractable industrial problems.

Buchman, aware that less and less people were attending church, knew they might go and see a play where they would not go to hear a sermon. Throughout the 19 years I was with him, he used plays as one of the chief public expressions of his philosophy and actions.

I had never thought of myself as an actor, or at least not since the days when we made that movie in Regina. But the part of the labour agitator seemed to fit my personality, and I was, so to speak, type-cast in the role. We had two professionals with us, Phyllis Konstam, Bunny Austin's wife, and Marion Clayton Anderson of Hollywood. They did their best to train us in articulation, how to move on stage, how to be natural, and the other details needed to make a performance convincing.

Another man I first met around the same time was called Peter Howard. He came with other British colleagues to Mackinac Island to meet Buchman at the end of the war in September, 1945.

He was a man of many parts – sportsman, farmer, husband

and father, author and journalist. To some he was a man of vision. To others he was a thorn in the flesh. But from the moment we met, we were friends.

He was a well-known British journalist, with a pen that had been feared in Fleet Street and far beyond. He had worked for Lord Beaverbrook on the *Daily Express*. During the war he came into contact with people from the Oxford Group and – as he later explained it – in an effort to get a scoop story about them, he went along to some of their meetings in London, saying the things he felt was expected of someone who might be interested in their work. What he hadn't expected was that his whole life's motivation changed, and drastically. His was an outstanding personality, and it was no small thing when he decided first to put his life under God's control, and then to throw in his lot with the men and women of Moral Re-Armament.

We acted in a few plays together – *The Dictator's Slippers*, which Peter had written; I played the dictator and Peter the prisoner. In *We are Tomorrow* which he also wrote, he played a man called Pewter, the Dean of a University College, and I was the college servant, 'Memory', who remembered only what suited him. I was a journalist named Fish in Peter's first play, *The Real News*.

He was lively – I remember at Mackinac seeing him doing his Christmas jumps, as he called them, when he would jump right off the ground, throw his legs out to one side and click his heels together before touching the ground again.

He possessed a tremendous sense of fun and humour – invigorating, irrepressible. His letters to me very often began, 'My dear old Paulus . . . .' and usually ended by signing off in all manner of unconventional greeting.

I played golf with him sometimes, and we played tennis – usually with Bunny Austin. Bunny remarked to us once that even at Wimbledon he had not experienced such fierce competition.

In 1945 I was with Buchman and his whole team at the San Francisco UN meeting. Then on to Britain on the Queen Mary, which was still fitted out as a troop ship, having been derequisitioned only hours before our tickets were applied for.

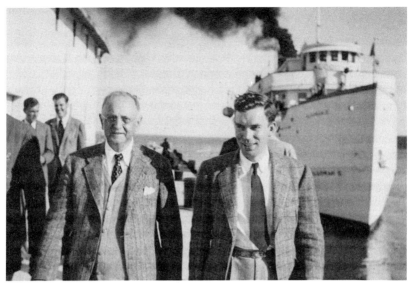

'Buchman was a merry soul. He had a mischievous twinkle in his eyes.'

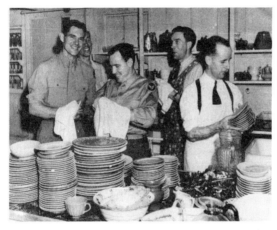

'The friendship and camaraderie were so infectious.'

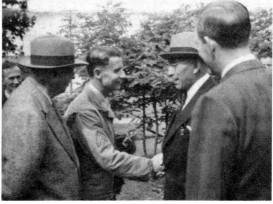

'Dad came to Mackinac in 1944, where he met many of my friends, including Buchman, Alan Thornhill and Bunny Austin, on leave from the US Air Force.'

The Forgotten Factor played to capacity audiences of coal miners in Doncaster, the Midlands, the Welsh coalfields and in Scotland. *The Spectator*, a well-regarded British weekly, in an article on this campaign, reported spectacular increases in coal production and the birth of a new spirit in the miners and their homes.

Buchman was fully aware of the reality and threat of materialism, whether it was of the Left with Stalin, the Right with Hitler and Mussolini, or the steely selfishness of the people in the West. He knew from rich experience that people can change and live honestly and unselfishly, whatever the cost. He had seen people changed in American and Canadian industries.

He also saw Communist operatives, steeped in 25 years of indoctrination, won to a moral ideology. There was the East London man, a militant agitator, sitting in the kitchen of his home, who was asked, 'Mr Keep, how does Communism work?'

Before he could reply, his wife put her head around the corner and said, 'I'll tell you, it works like hell around here!'

Men and women like that were quick to appreciate that a change in people is essential for a change in the system, otherwise human selfishness will pull down the best of structures. Buchman's faith was not in a movement but in the fact that even the most difficult person can be changed. And when people become different, situations, relationships and nations change.

Certain Swiss friends shared this faith. Four of them had come to confer with us on Mackinac Island, Michigan, where we were holding an assembly in 1945. On their return home they were able to purchase a disused resort hotel at Caux-sur-Montreux. It had been used by war refugees who had fled into Switzerland. 100 Swiss families, at great sacrifice, provided the resources to buy the property, Mountain House, from the bank which had scheduled it for demolition. These Swiss had the vision of what such a place could do to rebuild Europe and the rest of the world after the War, and the courage and tenacity to follow their dream.

I went with Buchman in the summer of 1946 first to Paris, where he met many old friends, and then to Switzerland. When he arrived at the door of Mountain House, at Caux, practically all the nations were represented. Buchman received their welcome, looked around and asked, 'Where are the Germans? You will not reconstruct Europe without the Germans.'

Keeping in mind that this was less than a year after the end of the Second World War, Buchman's simple statement was electric. Not many people had given creative thought to the future of the German nation.

But it was at Caux that the Germans were first received on equal terms after the war. They were the first of 7,000 Germans who in the next few years came to Caux, along with Italians, British, Americans, French, Dutch, Canadians, Australians and Japanese and Filipinos. People of many nationalities found changes in attitude – forgiveness and unity – through the application of absolute moral standards and the will to seek what is right not who is right as the principle on which to reconstruct a divided world.

In 1952 Buchman went to India, at the invitation of 18 senior men in Indian public life, with 250 people, four plays and some tons of stage equipment. The trip lasted seven months and was financed by generous gifts from convinced friends in many parts of the world. We had all ages with us, from teenagers to octogenarians, many of whom were in India for the first time. Not so Buchman, who had been there in 1915, when he had met Mahatma Gandhi.

It was hot, very hot. Buchman took good care of himself, wearing a wool cummerbund around his middle at night to prevent being chilled while the ceiling fans cooled the room. He was always careful to wear a sun helmet, and seemed to thrive in the heat.

I – medically speaking – had my hands full with the care of the large force of people, particularly with stomach complaints, skin rashes, acute headaches, scorpion bites and malaria.

We went to several cities – Calcutta, New Delhi, Madras, Bombay, Ahmedabad and Srinagar. One of the party, a press baron, produced a special edition of his Calcutta paper, given entirely to the work and philosophy of MRA.

Papers in Madras and Bombay also had special editions on Buchman and his battle for the world. Some Indians claim that it was the life and living of those visitors, with a spirit that knew no race or class boundaries, that began the swing of India at that time away from Moscow's gravitational pull, ensuring a democratic orientation.

Chapter Five
TWO-LEGGED LOCUSTS

THE VICTORY AT Dien Ben Phu which drove the French from Vietnam was a stimulus to dissidents in other French colonies. In August 1953 the Sultan of Morocco was deposed by the French and sent into exile in Madagascar. Barely a week later, terrorist action began in Morocco, with assassination an everyday affair. It was seen as an attempt to destroy the ability of France to rule, by eliminating the Moroccans on whom the French depended for the information that enabled them to exercise control over the Moroccan cities.

In September 1953, Robert Schuman, a former Foreign Secretary of France, came to the Caux assembly. He is one of the fathers of modern Europe, and a political personality in France who felt very concerned with the Moroccan situation.

At his suggestion, Buchman went to Morocco in February, 1954, taking five of us with him to Marrakech. One thing he hoped to do during his visit was to make contact with the family of El Glaoui, the Pasha of Marrakech, because he understood the vital nature of El Glaoui's rôle in the Franco-Moroccan crisis.

Marrakech is known for its large forest of palm-trees, which may well be one of the biggest in Africa. The city stands in the middle of a vast plain dominated by the Atlas Mountains. When we arrived in February this mountain wall had a covering of snow.

A French plantation owner, living about 20 km. from Marrakech, came to visit us. His name was Pierre Chavanne. A relative of his in France had told him about Buchman's visit, and urged him to meet us.

Pierre Chavanne and his wife Jeanine had two young children at that time, and a 300-hectare farm, employing 50 or so Moroccans in the plantations of orange, olive, apricot and almond trees. He had no faith, but after discussion with us he courageously agreed to experiment with listening to

51

the voice of Truth in his heart, just as I myself had done in Edmonton 20 years earlier.

In the summer of 1954 Pierre and Jeanine Chavanne visited the Caux assembly, and it was there that their lives underwent a fundamental change. Again the thought of listening to the deepest thing in his heart, and acting on it, came to the fore-front of Pierre's mind. However, as he had no far-reaching or concrete thoughts, when he experimented with a time of quiet reflection one morning at Caux, he decided to abandon his attempts.

It was at that moment that a very simple idea intruded into his mind. 'If you don't know where to begin to change yourself, ask your wife. She will have plenty of ideas.'

Without further ado Pierre asked his wife this question. And he asked it in such a way that Jeanine, though taken aback, realised she could genuinely say what she felt. Thus began a new chapter in their lives – a process of honesty and transparency which transformed their previously fragile relationship and created the climate in which a new and stronger one could grow. At the same moment faith in God was refound.

They decided to shape their lives by absolute moral standards – which translated in practical terms into the thoughtful care they gave the workers on the farm, in the way they made decisions as a family at home, and in their attitudes to the Muslim people of their host country.

In 1955 there was a locust plague in Morocco. The Department of Agriculture did an excellent job in killing the locusts before they could attack the trees and crops, and Chavanne's farm was saved from desolation.

One morning soon after, his waking thought was to go into the city, personally to thank the head of the Department of Agriculture for protecting his property so efficiently.

He found himself face to face with an energetic young man, Ahmed Guessous, who, unknown to Chavanne, was a member of the Istiqlal (Moroccan Nationalist) party. His avowed aim was to drive the French from his country. He was once giving a talk about the locust swarms to a group of French settlers and said, 'There is another type of locust, the one on two legs.' He was alluding to the French themselves, feeling that when they have come and gone, nothing is left.

When Guessous asked why he had come to see him, Chavanne spoke of his decision to apply absolute moral standards to his affairs. Guessous listened politely, but did not respond with much warmth. Yet his interest was caught, for, as head of the Department of Agriculture, he knew quite a bit about Chavanne's new and helpful relationship with his farmworkers.

A short time later Guessous invited Pierre and Jeanine Chavanne to dinner in his home. Jeanine was quite apprehensive as to what the evening might hold. Later the Chavannes discovered that Guessous was wary of the very notion that any Frenchman could deal in moral standards – fearing the authorities had sent Chavanne as a spy.

Guessous noted that his French guests did not drink the wine which, out of politeness, he had provided for them with the meal – even though as a Muslim he himself was forbidden to touch it. They explained to him that they had decided not to drink alcohol any more, as they felt it was an insult to their host country, and little more than an indulgence for themselves.

Gradually Guessous came to realise that there was a sincerity to Chavanne which he had not initially been ready to credit him with. The two families became friends, and frequent guests in each others' homes.

After a meal in the Chavannes' home, Ahmed Guessous remarked, 'There is an unusual spirit in this house – what is it?'

The Chavannes told him that, in the past, sometimes Pierre had tried to control the family affairs, and sometimes Jeanine, but that nowadays, together, they sought to find what was right on issues and plans, without control, pressure or manipulation.

A year later the bush telegraph, the 'téléphone arabe', circulated the story through the Marrakech souk that Pierre Chavanne had asked his Moroccan cook to help him destroy his remaining half-dozen bottles of liqueurs, because he and his wife had decided never again to serve alcohol in their home. As it happened, the story was true.

The young Nationalist, Guessous, was impressed by the

new attitudes he met in the Chavannes, and by what they told him of Frank Buchman's work of Moral Re-Armament. He agreed to go with Pierre to the Caux assembly then in progress.

Buchman asked me to chair the morning session of the conference on the day they arrived. There were 30 or 40 nationalities in the audience. The Moroccan flag had been hung at the front entrance, in honour of Guessous. And I spoke, with warmth, of our stay in Morocco, and the hospitality we had received at one of the castles of El Glaoui, whom I described as 'a powerful leader of South Morocco'.

At the end of the meeting Chavanne came to me, furious, exclaiming, 'You made one hell of a mistake this morning.'

Up came Guessous, whom I had never previously met – an extremely angry young man, with eyes flashing and voice trembling with rage. 'I came here thinking this was holy ground,' he said. 'But all you've done is talk about the Devil. The Glaoui of Marrakech is the Devil Incarnate. He is a friend of the French. If I'm to remain here another hour you must promise never to mention his name again in my presence.'

I invited him to sit down to lunch with me. He spent most of the meal pointing out where I had given a misleading impression of his country to the representatives of many nations. I kept thinking, 'What can I say to this man that will make any difference?'

My only thought was to say to him, 'In my own life I know I am no closer to God than I am to the person from whom I feel most divided.'

'What is that?' he asked, in surprise.

I repeated what I had said.

The young man put down his knife and fork and left the table. Later he told me that the idea went round and round in his head, and every time it came to the front, there was the image of El Glaoui, the feudal chief he hated.

'If I'm no closer to Allah than I am to El Glaoui, I'm a long way from home,' Guessous admitted to me.

This new insight which he gained during his visit to Caux stood him in good stead when he returned to Morocco. While he had been in Switzerland the violence in Morocco had escalated dramatically, beginning with the massacre of 49

French people, 15 of them children, at Oued Zem. The French army took terrible reprisals and violence erupted all over the country, leaving hundreds of Moroccans and many French dead.

Through Ahmed Guessous, Si Sadek, the son of El Glaoui, was in contact with the executive committee of the Istiqlal party, seeking ways to try and end the violence. I myself had met Si Sadek in the course of my visit to Marrakech with Buchman, when we had enjoyed a good game or two of golf together. He later became Chief Justice of Marrakech.

After three days of talks between Si Sadeq and the committee, a date was arranged for three of the Istiqlal men to meet El Glaoui himself. Guessous was one of the three.

If Ahmed Guessous had remained as aggressive towards El Glaoui as he had been when speaking of him to me at Caux, who knows if the talks would not have ended in deadlock? The fact that he went to the talks was in itself an acknowledgement of his own wrong attitudes of hatred. In European tradition it is customary to voice an apology in order for healing to begin. In the tradition of the peoples of North Africa, the very act of accepting to meet your enemy is a step taken in the spirit of forgiveness.

The meeting went well. Later the same day El Glaoui went to the Regency Council, established by the French to try to resolve the issue of the monarchy. There, in Rabat, El Glaoui dropped what is still referred to as 'the Pasha's bombshell'. 'I refuse to bring the loyalty of South Morocco to this Council,' he announced. 'I demand the return of the Sultan to his rightful throne.'

A few days later a picture reached the world through the press. It was of the Sultan, seated on a chair in a hotel on his way home to Morocco, reaching down to touch El Glaoui prostrate at his feet, in the customary attitude of one greeting his sovereign. The relationship was restored, and because of that I believe countless lives were saved.

Subsequently the Sultan wrote Buchman, 'You will find ready soil for your ideas here in Morocco.'

During the three month stay with Buchman in Marrakech I wrote a large section of a new book which I was working on with Peter Howard, entitled *Remaking Men*. It was published in 1954, and was translated in at least nine languages in the months thereafter. The dustjacket summed the book up as being about 'how to understand and redirect the most powerful forces in the human personality, and so to reconstruct the character of men and nations . . . it is a practical guide to the creative action every man can take to meet the conflicting tensions of the ideological age we live in.' Buchman's moral ideology was, and still is, sanity in an increasingly uncertain world situation.

Remaking Men was clinical in its approach to analysing and meeting the needs of individuals – but then I was trained, as a doctor, to use my mind that way. I was taught to analyse, diagnose and prescribe for cure. It is more than likely that it might have been written differently if I had, at that time, had a wife to offer comments and suggestions on the working manuscript.

Some have argued that the very tone of the book, its strong statements, the words chosen to express certain facts and deeply-held convictions, may have contributed to a climate of thought among some, a sort of corporate belief, which had more to do with fear of one's fellow-man than with the love of God. Likely some became more influenced by what so-and-so might think than by the simple tenet of 'thus saith the Lord'.

But it was during this same period that Buchman would gather his people together every morning in his room, to go over the day's plans, and I think the 'supranational cabinet', which he always hoped would come into being, began to have practical and realistic application. The men and women around him had to take up the task, with Buchman himself less able to do things personally, after his stroke.

It was a group of men and women all immensely talented in their own fields, who had thrown in their lot with Buchman. It was not surprising that at times we made mistakes, with so many of all ages, backgrounds and nationalities. Sometimes, also we lived in a kind of climate around Buchman where we almost disregarded our feelings, not spending time fussing about ourselves, but getting on with the very big job we felt called by God to do. That may or may not always have been a good thing.

Having said that mistakes were made, I have always felt

people should have the courage of their own convictions, and if they think something is wrong they should say so. It is all part of the growth and evolution of a spiritual work, and no one ever promised it would be easy.

In 1955 Peter Howard and my old friend from the Regina Camp, Cece Broadhurst, together wrote the lyrics of *The Vanishing Island*, a musical play of stunning quality and insight, for which George Fraser and William Reed wrote the music.

The World Mission, as the world tour of *The Vanishing Island* came to be known, included a group of distinguished men and women who made the journey alongside the theatre presentation, and who spoke after each showing, and at other meetings during the day. For Buchman, fond as he was of the theatre, a play was always only a means to an end – reaching nations with news of an answer.

In the event it was far too arduous an undertaking for Buchman himself, so he and a few others of us moved at a less demanding pace, and followed the travels of the Mission by letter and wire. Howard and company ran into considerable hostility in different parts of Asia, and from certain sections of the press who attempted to report falsely or to suppress reports on what had been happening. Howard tells the whole story in his book, *An Idea to Win the World*.

Howard wrote newsletters for Buchman of the visits of 'the Mission' to the various countries which had asked for it to come. He also wrote me with colourful asides, illustrations and insights.

(P D Howard to Paul)
July 1955, Pines Hotel, Baguio, Philippines,
(manager: A D Resurreccion)
My dear old Paulus,

You will enjoy the name of the manager of this hotel. In the same category as Suffering Moses of Kashmir. This *is* heavenly. Glorious skies and mountains – as cool as springtime (we even had a blanket over us at night) and a *wonderful* hotel where they charge us $5.50 (11 pesetas) a day, all found. Taiwan was tremendous. The Generalissimo's verdict to us was, 'Your visit has had a great effect not only here, but in the Communist countries. This is the most valuable form of aid we could have been sent.'

July 2nd, '55, Manila
My dear old Paulus,

Thank the Lord I've found a thicker piece of paper. The other stuff which Frank's is written on wilts in the heat. Your letter was such a joy, old friend, and a real help too – as some of the allusions in Frank's were a bit obscure to us. . . . The news from Mackinac refreshes us all. Brooks' words [the man who drove Buchman's carriage in Mackinac, where there are no cars] 'I did nothing . . . I was just there' are living truths for every would-be big shot in the world. . . . Ever as ever, Peter.

July 19th, '55, Connemara Hotel, Madras,
My dear old Paulus,

. . . . By the way, Frank's cable that the older people ought to be resting in the Nilgiri hills mysteriously reached us only this afternoon here in Madras. We have raised the point – but most of the older crowd seem to be full of pep and enjoyment. We are trying to care for them all. But when you see one senior man, beard streaming behind him – running, yes *running* and laughing at the same time, in this heat, what can you do?

August '55, Caux
My dear Paulus,

. . . . Did you see Krushchev's strong remarks about Geneva? It seems to me the man is right when he says that materialism organised into an ideology is not only stronger but more convincing than materialism disorganised and without one.

I think steadfastly of Frank. Let me know if there is any way I can help. . . . As ever, old friend, Yours, Peter.

November 6th, '55, Helsinki
My dear Paulus,

Just a couple of points to add to Frank's letter. In the

last three days we have had 850 inches of space in the three national newspapers. All seem to be 10,000% for us. Last night we were on the radio, which has a listening audience of two-and-a-half million people at that hour, and reaches an unknown multitude in the Soviet. . . . it took split-second timing, as the radio station is a quarter of an hour from the theatre and we had to get the quartet of singers etc. to and from the place while the play was running. All went well and people hit every cue in both places . . . My notebook is full of ideas for the book, but so far I've not squeezed an hour to write it down. It will come. . . . God gives us so much. Grateful for your friendship.

February 9th, '56, Bonn
My dear old Paulus,

Your magnificent letter of January 29th reached here today. You cannot imagine how convicted I feel when I see all the hard work you are doing! Seriously, I do rejoice at the progress of the book and am itching to get at it, but so far the itch seems everlasting.

. . . . . . I feel very much that we sometimes confuse giving a man faith with giving him corrective and though both are important they are not exactly the same thing . . . I simply pray God more and more to teach me how to live so that the men around me learn to feed only on God. One interesting point. While we were here the winner of the East German Peace Prize was allowed to speak at the University. His theme was simply: 'With your selfish ways you isolate yourselves from the great issues of the world. You know what you don't want. Do you know what you do want? That is the tragedy of the West.'

In 1955, when the World Mission returned to Caux, Buchman was there to welcome them. The assembly was in full swing, with over 900 participants, from at least 35 countries.

From Caux *The Vanishing Island* went to the main Swiss cities, then to Scandinavia. I accompanied Buchman straight to Italy, to Milan, where we were able to receive the cast when they arrived from the Nordic North. Alongside them was the African cast of the play *Freedom*, which had been written by a group of 29 Africans in three days at Caux.

In January 1956, 15 of us, including Prince Richard of Hesse, Bunny and Phyll Austin, Loudon Hamilton, whom I had first met at the 1937 Oxford house-party, and the Colwell brothers, a trio of talented American singers, set sail with Buchman from Genoa for Australia, arriving in Perth, and continuing by stages across the continent. When we reached New Zealand, Buchman disconcerted his hosts and those of us travelling with him by announcing he expected to stay for two years.

(PDH to Paul)
February 12th, '56, Bonn – (mailed to Australia)
My dear old Paul,

This brings you merry greetings from the polar bears of the frozen North. All this boasting and bragging of sunshine and calm seas is just plain cruelty to animals.

There was an interesting crowd in the theatre last night, which as usual was over-filled even to the window seats, and we took off the surplus in buses to an overflow meeting about a mile away skidding merrily through the snowdrifts and ice. Almost all the leaders of last year's uprising against the Communists in the East who have now fled to the West turned up at the play. They stayed talking till long after midnight . . . Their leader said, 'Last time we gained control for a day then they brought up the tanks. Next time there may be a breakthrough and the time after that there will be a breakthrough.' They certainly are some of the toughest, most courageous, and most ideologically hungry men I have ever met.

Frits Philips, the head of the Philips Electric Company of Holland, had offered to have a recording made of *The Vanishing Island* so that its truths and message could be even more widely available and heard around the world. We had to do the recording at night time because the studios were fully booked during the day.

Annejet, Frits Philips' daughter, began working full-time with MRA at the age of 20, and had travelled with *The*

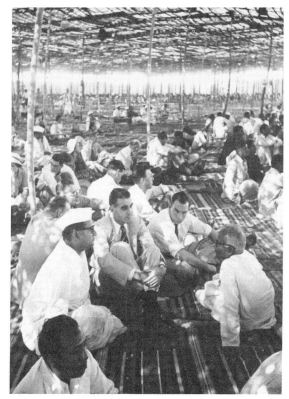

With Peter Howard in India, in 1952. Buchman took a party of 250 people with him, for a seven month visit.

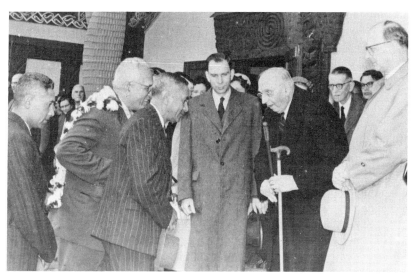

'When we reached New Zealand in 1956, Buchman disconcerted all of us in his party, and his hosts, by announcing he expected to stay for two years.'

Vanishing Island. She is a skilled dressmaker and designer, having learnt her art in Paris, and worked backstage on all the beautiful costumes the play required, creating and maintaining them.

(*PDH to Paul in New Zealand*)
March 9th, '56
. . . The recording of *The Vanishing Island* is now done. To my unskilled ear, it sounds a really superb job. After four nights work, from 11 pm to 7 am we heard the whole thing replayed – dialogue and all. Three places were not quite perfect, so we told the man whom Frits Philips had sent to do the recording that we would like to redo these bits tonight. He said it was not necessary and that he had to get back to Hamburg. Meanwhile Frits telephoned Annejet at the hotel, to know how we were getting on. He was really shaken and moved by the night work that all the crowd have so gloriously poured in. He said, 'We are going to have it absolutely perfect. We are going to distribute it to the world.' By the time Annejet had driven from the hotel to the radio station, Frits had already telephoned from Holland to the man and asked him to stay to complete the job.

I had visited the Philips home in Eindhoven, Holland, in 1948 on my way back to Caux with some of the large group Buchman took to tour Germany with the musical play *The Good Road*. I remember the lunch we had then, because the menu included fresh milk – an almost unknown commodity during our days in Germany.

I fell in love with Annejet Philips at Caux in 1954 while acting in one of Peter Howard's earlier plays, for which she was helping with the costumes. But I pushed away any idea of marriage, partly because I did not see how it could fit in with the life I led, with the care and attention Buchman required at all hours of the day and night. I was quite success-ful in my attempt to dismiss her from my heart and mind, at that time. Or so I thought.

Meanwhile in New Zealand, Buchman was becoming growingly uneasy about the perilous situation in the Middle East, and also at reports reaching him about *The Vanishing Island*, which at that time was playing to overflow houses in Britain. Nothing to be uneasy about in that, one might reasonably have thought – but Buchman perhaps felt his people were reporting rather too gleefully on the large crowds and queues waiting for tickets, and the successful speeches being made from the stage, rather than concentrating on meeting the needs of individual people one by one.

Whatever the reason, he startled those of us travelling with him yet again when he announced that he was going to 'hurry, hurry home'.

In the event we returned to Europe by way of Japan, Taiwan, the Philippines, Thailand, Burma and Iran – countries where the World Mission had been a few months before, to renew contacts with people there, some of them friends of 40 years' standing.

In Burma, for example, Buchman was asked by the Chief Abbot of Rangoon to write a message in the book kept at the top of the Golden Pagoda. He was not up to such an exertion and asked me to climb up and do it for him. 'What shall I write?' I asked him.

'Write that the next great moral and spiritual advance in the world will come from the East.'

Kichizaemon Sumitomo, a senior member of one of the great industrial families of Japan, said of Buchman, 'It is my great fortune to have met a man of such warmth and love. I have never known him say a joke that would hurt anyone, but the more you see of him the better you understand his care. I feel his prayers for me, that I become a new type of leader, not just in the Sumitomo concerns, but to contribute to the remaking of the world.'

As soon as he reached Britain Buchman spoke with those who were staging the successful showings of *The Vanishing Island*. He expressed his belief that large-scale results were very fine, but the programme of MRA needed to be securely founded on men and women who had decided to pay the price of full commitment to God's will in their own lives. With Peter Howard and other British colleagues he talked about the need for individual and personal work to be done with people who had been impacted by the play. Buchman did not intend to wound or depress his friends, but he longed to clarify and restore the depth of personal commitment to the life of his people.

This need for a Christ-centred life and health was something of which Howard was very aware, judging from letters he sent me around that same time.

However, by the summer of 1957 at Mackinac things came to a difficult stage. Buchman was forced by his state of health to keep mostly to his bed. There were those in his immediate, daily orbit who would try to relay to others what his thoughts and feelings were. Especially if he had spoken with some degree of heat or frustration, that tone of rebuke would likely be passed on to the next person, and so could easily be enlarged until the original point was lost in a cloud of accusation and hurt. Equally likely was the possibility that events, incidents or conversations were reported to Buchman at second- or third-hand, with a resulting loss of accuracy, and then he may well have spoken his mind on something which was not entirely true in the first place.

It was not an easy situation – his health prevented him from having personal contact with all the people at the assembly, and yet his sense of urgency meant he wanted to be sure that every single person was living in a way which would make the maximum difference to the world around them. But sometimes things went wrong.

Perhaps word got around that Buchman had been less than delighted with the last months of *The Vanishing Island* tour in Britain. At any rate, human nature being what it is, people looked for someone to blame, someone else to carry the can, so that they could save their own skins. To feel the full wrath of Buchman was not a pleasant experience – the more so, if he had a valid point.

There was a certain amount of singling-out, and of blame-apportioning – not so much by Buchman as by the people who were helping to run the assembly. Peter Howard stood head and shoulders above other colleagues – in his personality, clarity of conviction and articulate leadership. In Buchman's absence he had been one of the leaders of the World Mission. And at Mackinac that summer he was the target of some persistent criticism, even black-balling. He asked Buchman what to do, but I believe the only reply he received was, 'Go on doing what you have been doing.'

Howard felt finally that he had no option but to leave Mackinac, with his family. He returned to Britain, to his farm in Suffolk, completely at one with Buchman in his commitment, but isolated from some of the people around Buchman. It did not shake his life's direction, but I know it was very painful and costly for him and his family.

It was not till some months later that I began to realise how I had contributed to this state of affairs.

Chapter Six

BLESS YOUR BOOTS!

IN THE LATTER part of the summer of 1957 at Mackinac, Buchman felt I needed a rest. He was likely right. I not only looked after him by day and often many times during the night, but I took part in the meetings of the conference and in the plays, often as many as five separate productions in a weekend. I was sent to my room to rest.

My pride was somewhat damaged by the fact that I was thought to need a rest at all, so next morning I turned up for duty, saying I had had a good sleep. I was banished to my room again, to rest properly. I attended no meetings, played no theatre performances, had my meals in my room, took long walks around the Island, and slept a good deal for about two weeks. It gave me time to think also.

It was a summer when a lot of my friends were getting engaged – there were announcements seemingly every week. I went to congratulate one couple one evening.

'How about you, Paul?' they asked.

I replied that, with my responsibilities for the care of Buchman, I didn't see room for a wife in my life.

What I did not say was that I had kept thinking about Annejet Philips on and off over the past three years since I first fell in love with her, backstage at Caux. I had done my best to dismiss her from my heart and mind – at times with considerable success. It simply seemed preposterous to me, as long as I was Buchman's physician, to entertain the idea of adding a wife to the kind of life I lived.

However, the very next morning after greeting my newly-engaged friends, I had the thought that I should meet Annejet and tell her how I felt about her. Preposterous or not, it was an idea that, deep inside me, I longed for – so much so that I actually felt it was perhaps too good to be true, and that it might have been wishful thinking. To say that I was astonished at having such a thought is an understatement of considerable proportion.

I told Buchman what was on my mind. Later that day he returned to the subject with me. 'I'm not sure about your idea,' he said.

I was disappointed, because what Buchman felt about things carried a certain amount of weight with me. But on the other hand his caution about it helped me to sit loose to the whole idea. I felt my responsibility for his care too much to act on such a matter without his concurrence. What Annejet herself felt, I had no idea.

It was not till later that she told me what her own feelings had been, during that summer when there seemed to be engagements or weddings every single Saturday. She was very often involved, because of her dress-making skills, with fixing someone's wedding veil, or the hem of a wedding dress, and such matters.

One day, while working in the costume room of the theatre it all got a bit much. She said to herself, 'Everyone else is getting married and nobody's going to marry me.' Then, she got down on her knees, on the costume-room floor, and prayed, 'All right, God, I will trust you about all this.' She was 23.

A few evenings later I was at dinner with a delegation to the Mackinac assembly from Taiwan, when I had a message that Buchman wanted to see me. I found him in his sitting-room overlooking the lake. It was a beautiful evening, the moon reflected on the water. His first words were, 'I don't know why I had that hold-up on your thought to propose to Annejet. Do you still think it is right?'

I most certainly did, and said so.

'Then you must do it!' Buchman responded, whole-heartedly. I approached the whole possibility with a new sense of freedom, which was perhaps partly the result of having been willing not to propose, if that was what God wanted of me.

Annejet's parents, Frits and Sylvia Philips, were at the assembly at that time. He was then President of the Philips Electrical company, with some 320,000 employed around the world. I was conscious of the need to do things properly, so I invited them to tea the next afternoon. I told them of my thought about Annejet.

Her mother looked at me carefully, and in a slightly questioning voice remarked, 'I suppose he could make her happy?'

She was perhaps thinking of our very different backgrounds, and also of the fact that I was 45 – more than 20 years older than her daughter.

Her father, on the other hand, offered to go and fetch Annejet straight away, so I could speak to her then and there!

In the event, we hatched a less precipitate scheme. They asked Annejet to join them that evening in their suite and arranged for me to 'drop in'. At which point they both excused themselves.

I told Annejet the thoughts I had about our future, adding that she could take 10 minutes, an hour, a day, a month or a year to give me an answer. For her it was a bolt from the blue and, not knowing quite what to say, she very sensibly said she needed time to think.

But late the next evening, while brushing her teeth before going to bed, she had a crystal-clear thought. 'Paul is the man for you. Say "yes, with all my heart and gladly".'

Next day Frits Philips came up to me and asked if I would care to go for a walk with him by the lake. I was a little surprised, as it was raining at the time, but thought it best to do as he asked. When we got out of the door, there a little way in front of us, also in the rain, were Annejet and her mother. I don't recall how, but the parents melted away, and there was Annejet saying to me, 'Yes, with all my heart and gladly.'

So taken aback was I by this longed-for and yet scarcely-to-be-hoped-for response that I blurted, romantically, 'Bless your boots!' So, we became engaged, on September 11th. A senior Canadian couple, long-standing friends, gave me a ring to present to my future wife. It was a generous gesture, and one I greatly appreciated, as I had no money of my own with which to buy her a ring. My announcement that we had decided to travel the road together took friends at the assembly by surprise. Apart from the fact that our engagement bridged a generation gap, I think I may well have been regarded as a confirmed bachelor.

Annejet and her parents left shortly after our announcement to fulfil a long-standing engagement in Detroit, with the Henry Fords, whom Frits Philips knew. They had dinner in the Ford home, and then returned to Mackinac. Buchman was keen to know how it had gone, what had been said and by whom.

There was a large tea-party in one of the salons at Mackinac, with about 50 or 60 people. Buchman, as usual, asked different ones to tell the whole group such news as they had – 'messages from Japan', and so on.

Then he said, 'Now, Annejet, you've just been to Detroit, and you had dinner with Henry Ford, and what happened?'

She was unprepared, and stumbled through a short and vague account. She felt totally out of her depth and had not really thought about it from Buchman's point of view. He would be intensely interested to know what had taken place because he had known old Henry Ford and his wife Clara.

At the end of the afternoon, when most people had left, Frank took her to task and – as she told me later that evening – said to her, 'Now, look here. You're going to get married to Paul and he is like a son to me, and I want to make sure that you are going to live the life and not drag him down to your level.'

That night I met a considerably upset Annejet who had been deeply shaken by Buchman's words. She told me she understood what he was getting at – all through that time she had been content to. do her work with the costumes and the plays, and had been equally willing to leave larger responsibilities to others. Frank's words made her acutely aware that a more profound accepting of her calling was needed.

The wedding date was already set for October 5th – only about three weeks off – at Mackinac. Annejet's mother had rushed home to Holland to get the family lined up, invitations printed etc. With hindsight, a year later, we felt we would have been better to wait until the following spring to get married, but I think one thing that may have influenced me was that I had figured out Buchman's programme – which was of necessity also my own programme – and thought that if we didn't get married then and there, perhaps we never would – you never knew where Buchman was going to be next.

Annejet herself told me later, when the subject was open for discussion, that when we became engaged some people started to treat her differently, because she was my fiancée and they were in awe of me, as she put it. She acknowledged this to be a not unpleasant experience, being associated with someone whom others looked up to, for whatever reason. She also realised later that she had taken me totally for granted, in that she felt I had been with Buchman for umpteen years and must know things a lot better than she did. Life with me has, I think, rid her of that notion, but at the time she never even questioned the wedding date, although it was so sudden.

After her tea-party encounter with Buchman she had promised herself she would behave immaculately, so that no one would stop us from getting married. It was a subconscious thought, but a strong one.

In fact, Buchman himself posed a question which indirectly should have prompted us to reconsider the wedding date, but I was so hell-bent on our plans that I wouldn't have listened to anybody. He asked whether it was possible for Annejet's family to come so soon from Holland. Also, his health was not at all good at that point and I was, after all, his physician.

However, within a few short weeks we were married, and it was a glorious event. The ceremony took place in the Great Hall at Mackinac, and was performed by the Rev Alan Thornhill of England, and Bishop Bengt Jonzon of Sweden. There were at least 600 people attending the assembly at the time, and they were all invited to the wedding. Many of Annejet's family from Holland were present, including her parents, her maternal grandmother, her three sisters and three brothers, and various cousins, aunts and uncles.

Buchman had been due to be my Best Man, but on the actual day he was not feeling well and I advised him not to take part. Bunny Austin acted on his behalf. Archie Mackenzie, an old friend who was on the diplomatic staff of the British Foreign Office, gave the address. As the ceremony finished the Marquis of Graham played the bagpipes and led us down the aisle. After the official photos, we had a sit-down dinner for all the guests.

Buchman had heard the service over an intercom in his bedroom, and we went to see him afterwards. Though unmarried himself, Buchman offered us a piece of advice which we have found to be priceless – 'no secrets, no fights and no bluffing'. It has given our marriage a solidity and a unity which we prize.

Then we set off on October 6th, in a snowstorm, on a wedding trip to the Canadian West. We visited my Dad, who had not been able to come to the wedding. He took her straight to his heart.

At the end of a meal with him in a restaurant, I got up to pay the bill. While I was away from the table, Dad pushed something into Annejet's hand. It turned out to be a $50 bill, his wedding gift to us. For a retired pastor, in his circumstances, it represented a fabulous sum, and it moves me still when I think of it. We were very touched by his generosity, so typical of him.

We had 10 days in Canada, four of them in Banff, in those glorious Rocky Mountains, and then we returned to Mackinac Island.

Buchman was not well, and it had been long-planned that he and I and one or two others would winter quietly in a friend's house in Miami, Florida, to give him a chance to convalesce and regain his strength. At the same time, the main focus of our MRA programme in America that winter was the creation and staging of the play *The Crowning Experience*, about the life of Mary McLeod Bethune, the black teacher who founded the Bethune-Cookman College and rose to become adviser to the President of the United States. Annejet was committed to working on the costumes for this production.

So, there we were, engaged and married within a month, and then within less than a month we were separated. Many many times in the 34 years since then we have been living or working in different places. But somehow, in those early months, any demand in us to be always together was broken. It is hard to be apart, of course, but those experiences have built a certain flexibility, strength and independence into our union – and we are going stronger than ever.

There is a real joy in our lives, coming out of a frankness about what we feel and think, about our care for people and where it can be heightened, and all salted with a sense of humour that has us laughing together a great deal.

The other thing about being apart at frequent intervals is that Annejet has kept letters which I have written to her, through the years, and they give a vivid picture of people and events and insights of the time.

October 31st, 2.15 pm on a train en route to Miami

This may reach you Saturday, in time for our fourth week's celebration. We are passing through sub-tropical country now, with palm trees, orange groves and mis-shapen ladies in shorts playing at golf!

. . . Frank has had a very good journey – but is feeling slightly the unaccustomed exertion of the past 48 hours. He certainly is a very great deal better than on our return from the West . . .

Wednesday, November 3rd, 6.40 pm

What a joy to hear you on the phone. There was a lot of noise at this end – the house is having additions made to it – an elevator at the moment – I ended in a bathroom with all doors closed so I could hear you! I believe we are being prepared and tempered like steel for a matchless service together – and we need this breaking of being run by what we want right at the beginning of our life together I have lived so much by by-passing my feelings I need all your help to even know what I am feeling. For the moment we are sort of camping out with the building going on – and the cottages to be fixed up etc.

Thursday, 4 pm, November 7th

This was the day we motored from Edmonton with Dad, had lunch with the Muirs. And you will receive this on Saturday, our 5th week! . . . You remember our visit to the Ben Hawkins' home. It suddenly struck me I was so proud I resisted just a bit your seeing how simply Dad lives, and yet was really glad that you had.

Mitch [the friend who loaned Buchman his house in Miami] was in last night and said he had always thought of Frank being surrounded by dominating personalities (!) – But that our marriage was making it more the spirit of a family. . . . he may have a point there.

The hammering and sawing continues noisily. Now

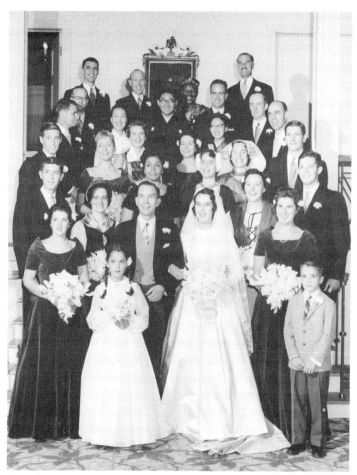

'Annejet and I were married on October 5th, 1957, and it was a glorious event.' Many of Annejet's family were present, and 600 delegates at the conferences, among them those who, with Annejet, were undertaking the production of *The Crowning Experience*, including Muriel Smith and Ann Buckles.

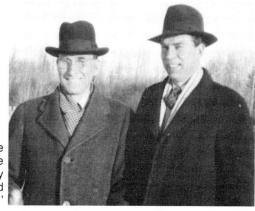

'Dad had a rare spirit. He completely trusted God and loved him.'

they are going to build a porch outside Frank's window so he isn't cramped inside four walls all the time.

Remember that prairie harvest moon coming out of the ground?

Friday, 6.15 pm
My dear Mrs Campbell

Remember me? The fellow you went to Banff with four weeks ago today! What a day.

Frank is far from well since yesterday afternoon so I was up a lot in the night and on constant watch during the day. He is picking up again tonight. But it is not very easy or comfortable for him. He just said he had several bouts like this (rapid pulse and exhaustion) while we were away. This time it's due I think to some medicine he was given for the lungs, which can upset the heart a bit . . . I got a short five-minute walk down the street this afternoon in the cool of the setting sun. It has been very sultry these past two days. I was looking for the walks we can take when you come.

During those months I and another friend, Jim McLennan, took it in turns to sleep next door to Buchman's room, in case he needed help in the night. Three nights on and three nights off.

(P to A)
Sunday

Frank is a bit better today – I know you will be praying for him. Jim has been up more at night with him than I have, and yesterday instead of encouraging him to sleep I let Jim go out. So Frank said to me this morning, 'You are a hard task-master. Not everyone has your iron constitution.' I apologised to Jim for my lack of care for him.

. . . Earlier this morning I had this thought, 'Tremendously grateful for Annejet's commitment. It has freed me . . . and taken away all sense of separation.'

Sunday

Just 15 minutes ago I heard your voice in my ears.

There was a lot of noise at our end with two planes going over – but I could hear you. I didn't want to talk too loud and waken Frank . . . who had the usual night. I was with him at 10.30, 12.00, 1.00, 2.20 when he had mint tea and pretzels! 4, 4.30, 5, 6, 7 – he often feels too hot and perspires a lot so I change his pyjamas, or he is too cold and needs more covering, or the room ventilated differently. I slept well between each call, and rested most of this morning. He looked better at breakfast time but by lunch time was not feeling well and ate sparingly. This afternoon we shall give him a tub-bath if he is up to it.

I am deeply concerned over Frank. There actually has been no basic improvement. He could of course surprise us all and rise up in new strength, but it will be a miracle. I am suggesting to a group of friends we enlist personalities who have had experiences with Frank to write them down. I believe his life will speak more and more loudly to this nation . . . he is an American with an answer recognized by the African, the Asian, the communist and the free-world materialist.

The other day he asked after you and said, 'You have been away from her a long time. I hope soon you will be able to go to her.' I was grateful for his thought for us, while he is far from well. Most men would be thinking only of themselves. None of us is indispensable – but right now I come close to it – for he needs a certain medical knowledge in administering his care which includes injections – as well as watching constantly the effect of the medicines he takes by mouth.

. . . Golly, I miss you, but can have peace and joy at the same time that we are the children of God's matchless and perfect care.

Sunday morning

These have been of necessity very painful hours for me as God has made frightfully clear the cost of myself to you, Frank, and the whole fellowship, and most of all to the Lord Himself . . . . I have a life-long habit of repressing uncomfortable conviction and keeping quiet about it.

The Lord gave us a glorious wedding and a wedding

trip of superb perfection. But I have the strong conviction that for your sake and mine I pushed the wedding date too fast. I didn't wait for the Lord's timing. Actually the Lord tried to speak through Frank's condition and physical needs, but I wouldn't listen. I rebelled against a lengthier engagement which is actually what we both needed – to get to know each other better and to find the freedom from each other which puts the Lord in control. I precipitated you into a position which had the opposite effect on us both. . . . I need to be like a boy shaken by the heels till all the hidden and forgotten junk in the pockets comes out on the carpet – and stay that way. That's what's happening now. . . . I pray for you constantly and all those you are with. You have brought to focus in my life all those things which would still be hidden. Grateful to the Lord and you – with all my heart.

I also realised that I owed a long-overdue apology to Peter and Doë Howard, since the difficult days when they felt they had to leave Mackinac earlier that summer. I wrote to them at Hill Farm, Suffolk.

(Paul to PDH and Doë)
Autumn '57, Miami,
 . . . . I have real restitution to make to you both for the cold self-righteousness of my dishonesty, pride and self-protection. It has been anything but 'unfeigned love of the brethren'.

Ambition for place and prominence were my real motives in working with you. When I felt you could no longer give me these I dissociated myself from you – and left you at the cold end of the accusing finger. . . . My own skin has always come first.

I weep when I think of the cost . . . . Apology is not enough. It's got to be the Cross in my own heart in every relationship from now on. I cannot calculate the cost to others, but I do feel the pain of it.

Peter replied, writing on the morning of his and Doë's 25th anniversary, in mid-Dec.:

Your letter was a landmark in life. It struck deep to the heart.

(P to A)
Thanksgiving Day, end November '57
We've just come up from a magnificent turkey dinner. It was Frank's first meal downstairs in 24 days – a marking event. 15 years ago in Saratoga, on Thanksgiving Day, he made his first turn for the better following his stroke . . .

I woke with tremendous joy this morning – and was praying for the mind and heart to live in the magnitude of God's will and power for the nations . . . . It suddenly struck me today that I'm very concerned of what you think of me. And I saw that that is the basis of wife-pleasing and man-pleasing in general. . . . Our love for each other will deepen and broaden and heighten day by day. But at times in my heart has been the nagging fear that because of what I'm like – and our age difference – you might cease to care. Consequently there has been human demand in me that you should care – and it has tied me to real concern of what you think . . . The Lord said that whether you care or not is not my responsibility – but God's! The point is I must be free of demand that you do . . . .

This comes on our eighth week. I woke this morning grateful for my parents and the heritage they gave me, and above all grateful for you.

December 11th, '57
. . . We hear it is eight degrees below zero at Mackinac tonight with crunchy snow. My – how I'd like to be there.

Had a rough night again last night with Frank, with some improvement today, thank the Lord. I was up almost every half hour, so today I slept about an hour-and-a-half both before and after lunch.

Friday evening, 11.30 pm, Miami
This is one of our evening chats about the day. . . . I had a talk on the phone with our specialist this morning

and this evening his assistant came around. He's fairly gruff – as many young doctors trained in America are (!). Frank got up into a chair for half an hour to greet Mme Eboué, the French Senator. She is in good form – absolutely in raptures about her time with you all in Mackinac. She at first didn't realise I was the husband of the Mrs Campbell she had supper with on Sunday!

December 21st, '57, Miami.

. . . This morning Frank was all for going down town for a haircut – but discretion won the day! But he is feeling better. Jim and I are able to manage alright so far. Good news in from Rome today will be a real tonic to Frank's spirit, and worth many bottles of medicine! He was out of bed for tea and dinner yesterday. He says it's amazing how God pours energy in.

Lucy Clark, whom you ask about, is an old flame of mine – in fact she's about 70, Frank and a few of us lived in her home in Los Angeles for three different winters. Her father put down the street railways in LA . . . She had some prize glass – gold-inlaid goblets – brought out for special occasions. We did the wash-up under her beady eye when the goblets were being done. Reg Sheppard was helping once. She asked, 'And what do you do, Mr. Sheppard?' 'Oh,' said Reg, as he put his big mit on a goblet, 'I'm a hard-rock miner.' Poor Lucy nearly collapsed. I'm delighted she remembered us.

Christmas Eve, '57, 6.30 pm

This morning Morris [Martin] and I visited the doctor's offices with calendars and quarterly magazines, giving news and reports of MRA's programme, for everyone – including the two receptionists, the coloured girl who does odd jobs, the two girls who run the elevators and the men in the drug store, as well as the doctor's professional associates. Then we visited the hospital where Frank was operated in '52. They were really overjoyed to see us.

Frank had his mail read – or rather part of it. He cannot take too much at a time. I was exhausted last night, slept every time I hit the pillow which was every hour and a half from 9.00 pm till 7.30 am – yet wakened every time he switched on his light or coughed. He never has to call me – I waken first. I wonder if he will have the energy for midnight mass tonight.

This afternoon two of the boys brought a beautifully decorated tree – table-size for Frank's room. It has the tiniest electric lights I've seen – Frank loves it.

. . . It came to me today – real purity is simply loving the other person more than yourself. It is a positive, not a negative. And loving you more than myself – is that not the meaning of the Christmas Babe?

Annejet joined me in Miami in January, 1958, and we had four months together there until the Mackinac assembly started in May. Buchman was really not at all well that winter, with cardiac trouble, and then pneumonia. It was a different world for Annejet, away from the rather glamorous world of the theatre – instead she was learning how to do the laundry, wash the dishes and look after the guests who came frequently. But it was a wonderful gift to be together.

Chapter Seven

THE BEST CRAP GAME

WHILE BUCHMAN, Annejet and I and a few others remained quietly in Miami in the early part of 1958, the play *The Crowning Experience* was staged for five months in Atlanta. Muriel Smith, a black mezzo-soprano of great talent, took the leading role in the play, and Ann Buckles, fresh from Broadway, co-starred. At a time when riots over the colour issue were daily national news, we had a mixed-race cast of an MRA musical play giving public performances to multi-racial audiences in the American South. It was the first time in that Atlanta theatre that the different races were allowed to enter the auditorium through the same door.

On June 4th, 1958 Buchman was to celebrate his 80th birthday on Mackinac Island. He made plans early, because he wanted to have all his old friends invited, anyone who fitted into that category.

Someone suggested it would be appropriate to invite Chief Walking Buffalo of the Stoney Indians of Alberta to be present. Walking Buffalo was the man who, in 1934 at Banff, Alberta, had made Buchman a Blood Brother of the Stoney tribe, naming him 'Great Light in Darkness'. Till then the only white people to be accorded such an honour had been members of the British Royal Family.

Buchman seized eagerly on the idea, and asked one of his friends, Ken McCallum from Calgary, to go find Walking Buffalo, and invite him to come to Mackinac. This was easier said than done, for the old man was often away from home, horseback riding in the Rocky Mountains.

In the meanwhile, another person recalled that, at the ceremony in 1934, Buchman had been given a beautiful buckskin outfit, with feathered bonnet, moccasins, and the full regalia. Perhaps, she suggested to Buchman, it would be fitting for these gifts to be displayed in the Great Hall at

81

Mackinac – a huge room made of wood in the shape of an enormous teepee.

Immediately Buchman put the matter in hand – sending messages to England to find the trunk containing his Indian regalia, which was stored in someone's attic; to find the key for said attic and said trunk, and ship the whole lot to him at Mackinac Island.

Walking Buffalo was eventually found, somewhere in his loved mountains, and accepted to join Buchman in June. The trunk and regalia were found and despatched by ship from England – and arrived in the Great Hall with just time enough for the buckskin outfit to be pinned to the wooden wall of the Great Hall 'teepee' barely an instant before Walking Buffalo and his party were ushered in and welcomed.

It was a moment of magic – the old man recognized the gifts he had given Buchman almost a quarter of a century earlier, and it touched him to see them displayed thus.

Buchman insisted that Walking Buffalo be given the best guest-room in the place. Likely the Chief would have been more comfortable in a room more akin to his one at home, but he recognized that he was being treated as a Chief, by a Chief. He stayed at Mackinac for three weeks, and in those three weeks he lost his bitterness against the white man.

Every day Buchman offered him the chance to speak to the assembly. Some days he would pull everyone's legs, with his matchless sense of humour. Other days he would almost spill over with some of the degrading things that had happened to him – like the time when he was on a train and one person after another of the whites in the carriage got up and moved down the train, until he was all alone. He told us what it was like to be photographed day after day for his regalia by tourists, none of whom spoke to him or looked him in the face, or in any way treated him as a human being. He spoke about the people who brought liquor to the Native people – 'they were the real barbarians,' he said.

There were 800 people at that assembly, and every day the Chief was listened to. One day, towards the end of his stay, the chorus sang from the platform, where he was also sitting. They stood in their colourful national costumes and sang for him, 'Take the spirit of the West where'er you go . . .'

Partway through the song the Chief, who had previously

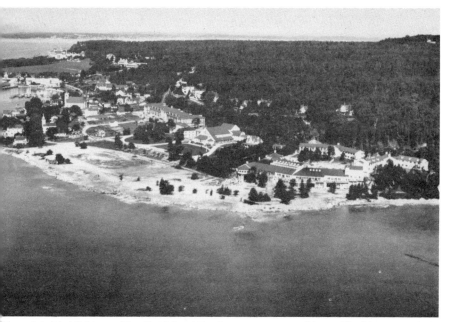

kinac Island, Michigan. The first Moral Re-Armament assembly on Mackinac was held
disused hotel, renovated for the purpose, and rented for the sum of $1 a year. Further
erence buildings were added and the Island was host to MRA assemblies for over 20
s.

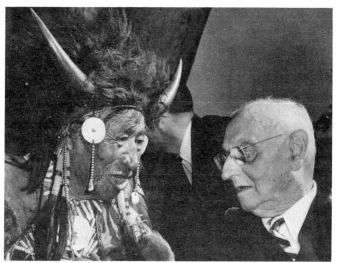

Chief Walking Buffalo attended Buchman's 80th birthday
celebrations in 1958.

been a rather bent old man, stood up, ramrod straight, with his medicine stick in his hand, and remained at attention till the song finished. He never walked bent over again. Someone said it was as if he was flinging off the robes of bitterness – after those three weeks of being asked to say everything that was on his heart, and being listened to.

From Mackinac he went to Washington, to be present at a performance of *The Crowning Experience*. He also visited Hollywood sometime later, when the film of the play was shown there. A woman journalist came up to him in the auditorium, and said, 'If I may say so, Mr. Buffalo, you do look frisky!' – meaning to compliment him, on hearing his age.

The Chief replied with the glimmer of a smile, 'I never drink whisky.'

Thinking he had misheard her, the woman repeated her remark, only louder. 'I said, you do look frisky!'

Again the Chief responded, 'I don't drink whisky.'

After the woman's third attempt the Chief relented and said, 'I look frisky because I don't drink whisky!' It must have given her something to think about at her next cocktail party.

Later in the summer, after returning to Canada, Chief Walking Buffalo made a second visit to Mackinac with members of his family, and people from other tribes of Southern Alberta. Among them were Chief David Crowchild and his wife Daisy, and their sons Gordon and Arnold, who later became two of my very good friends.

In November 1958 Buchman and I and a small party went to Tucson to spend the winter in the kinder climate of Arizona. Once again, Annejet remained in Mackinac, where they were filming *The Crowning Experience*. Among other things she had to make 24 hats for a scene in the exclusive Washington Ladies' Club. During that time I gained new insight into my own life. Peter Howard was a true friend, in the way he gave me corrective when he felt I needed it. He really managed to set me thinking.

(Paul to PDH)
November 10th, '58, Tucson
   I was really touched by your letter. . . . Achievement

has been my security and failure the worst thing that could happen to me – so when corrective came I got bitter. I always prided myself on being too magnanimous for that. But I get revenge by withdrawal, by a cruel refusal to give. It throws a severe burden on others and robs my friends of what God could give them through a humble and willing spirit. . . .The one thing I want is that God should lead – but in actual practice it has often been my will.

. . . The truth is I've judged almost everything by its effect on my desire for fame – the temptation which Jesus resolutely put behind him. He called it 'tempting God'.

For the last months I've done a lot of stewing around. I've been so self-centred that I've had no eyes for the Cross – the one source of life and health and peace. I've talked so much of faith and all the while lived by my own abilities and ideas. God has gloriously promised a new era in my life. . . . I ask your help and prayers not only to be different, but to stay that way. Thank you for writing the way you did.

(P to A)
November 12th, '58
I did Frank's meals on Monday, and did Monday night as well. Blanton Belk (bless his heart) did last night.

. . . I am learning I always need to temper my convictions with real love or else they just divide instead of winning and challenging. Directness with genuine selfless continuing care seems to be the answer. . . . Grateful for your fighting heart.

(P to A)
December 28th, '58
I thought of you a lot today, particularly this evening when showing *The Crowning Experience* Christmas photo-book to a young man and his wife who came in for supper. There you were – just made it at the edge of the page!

. . . Frank has stayed in bed the past 48 hours, resting from his Christmas exertions. But he's very well . . . .

This past year has been the richest of my life.

February 16th, '59

Frank is still quite tired and has not been up quite so much, but he is as sharp as a cactus needle and his memory is unfailing.

... The lady you mention in your letter sounds like one of those Christians who think anything they don't fully understand must be subversive! I'm like that myself! My first reaction to an idea which doesn't suit me is to reject it. But I'm learning – Frank always amazes me the way he entertains every suggestion.

The Hallwards have arrived here for a visit. You remember them – they gave me your engagement ring. At their first two meals I helped serve the table. And as I approached the second meal I suddenly thought, 'Will they think I've been demoted?' Which revealed two things at least – first I must think I had a position from which I could be demoted, and second that whatever that mythical position was it had more honour and prestige than comes with serving! It just shows how upside-down my values have been. For so long I've had an exaggerated idea of my own importance and place that I automatically expect consideration .... I'm such a proud fellow – I'd rather volunteer to do something like serving the meal, than be told to do it!

Tucson, '59

The more I trust God the less I trust myself, and the more I value God the less I value myself. With any kind of man-pleasing still alive in me Frank's encouragement can inflate me like a balloon. We need constantly a sane estimate of ourselves. A pin-prick is better than a sledge-hammer, of course, when it comes to dealing with balloons. There's a balloon in every man, and I believe every woman needs to know how to use the hat-pin effectively!

February 21st, '59

Yippee! We are all full of cowboys and rodeo here. On Thursday we went to the Annual parade, leaving the house before 9.00 am, then we went on to the rodeo, getting home by 6.30 pm. It was nine-and-a-half hours in the open air for Frank with only sandwiches for lunch! And how he enjoyed it. We had perfect weather and are all showing the reddening effect of pale-face exposure to the Southern sun. It was great fun.

The parade was very good with many examples of the old frontier stages, covered wagons, fire-engines, all horse-drawn, and of course an endless array of magnificent horses.

We had seats on the grandstand right at the road-side, only 15 yards from a school where we were able to have all the facilities we needed. During the parade Frank suddenly decided to go to the rodeo! This was unexpected. He said, ' . . . and I will take my car-load with me' – that was six of us altogether. We already had one box but didn't know how, at that late stage, to secure places for the rest of the party. Within a few minutes Blanton ran into an official who had been celebrating (he had a bar in the trunk of his car) – he said, 'Take my box', which we did, best seats in the house!! You would have loved it. The whole thing was very well done – bronco-busting, steer-wrestling and roping, Brahmin bull-riding; clowns, trained dogs, and gymnasts doing acrobatics on horse-back.

Frank is feeling the effect of it, and no wonder. He has done nothing like that for three years.

During our stay in Tucson many visitors came through from California, where an MRA assembly was taking place, to spend some time with Buchman. It was a most creative few months.

(P to A)
Friday, April 3rd, '59
The Japanese students left here all fired up and with a clear picture of what has to be done and with the unity to do it . . . Yesterday we read the script for the new South American movie. I think it has the makings of something very good. Today we go over the details of

The Crowning Experience film script. Peter and I are developing ideas for a book which could be a humdinger. This is the month to do it if it is to be done.

... Frank was saying the other day to the Japanese, 'What keeps me free of evil thoughts? Think of the magazines and books the people in Japan read all the time – so what do you need? If you want to be clean in your thought-life, get out and deal with people. The Holy Spirit can give you power to keep you from thinking of those things. If you're not winning you're sinning.'

Monday, April 6th, '59

Yesterday afternoon we had a remarkable party for the milk-man and the Western Union people, the egg-man, and the plumber. Said the milk-man, 'You couldn't be doing this for money. It must be that you really care for the world.' The ice-cream man's wife, after 23 years, had taken off with another man. He was in tears and resolved to write her and be honest with her about something she had not known. The 16-year-old son came with the father. One woman, who runs a food store, said she would remember the afternoon as long as she lives.

I was very grateful for you this morning, when I was thinking about you. 'Grateful for her commitment, bedrock and single-minded. We have only one "right" in life, to obey the Holy Spirit. He knows best and loves us the most.'

April 20th, '59

Hi darling – it's a glorious morning. I was on duty with Frank last night and so got a 4 am start on the day – which is not unusual around here. Just had some time with Frank . . . If the quality of commitment in people around us is not deepening it means we are not living it. Then we try as compensation to do for people what only God can do.

There is more to it than being direct and firm with people – that can be self-importance. Any time we become masters of a situation we develop 'a following' and do less than the maximum.

Today we welcome U Nu and his friends. Some of the Japanese remained on for the visit and will serve a Burmese curry to our guests.

The short-notice visit of U Nu, then Prime Minister of Burma, was part of Buchman's extraordinary range of long-term friendships. He treated every person exactly the same – the man who brought the milk and the eggs, the militant East London docker, or the Asian Prime Minister. For each there was the same detailed thought and planning.

The day before U Nu arrived in Tucson, the whole menu for the Burmese meal that was to be served was prepared and served to Buchman and his household, to make sure there would be no mistakes on the day.

After the Prime Minister came in, Buchman caught sight of some men outside, standing around in front of the house. They were U Nu's American police motorcycle escort. Buchman insisted they be brought in to meet U Nu. One cop remarked afterwards, 'That was the best crap game I've ever been in.'

Buchman and U Nu remained friends for many years, keeping contact through letters.

April 25th, '59

. . . These last days have been fabulous. At 4.45 the other morning Frank began on letters to all corners of the earth – Emperor Haile Selassie, U Nu, Saragat, Queen Helen, Henry Ford, Gabriel Marcel, President Tubman, Dr. Azikiwe of Nigeria, the Tolon Na of Ghana, William Nkomo of South Africa, Marinotti. They are all being invited to a summit strategy conference in Mackinac.

. . . Dear old Dad has forgotten my birthday for the first time. I sent him the story about U Nu, and the miracles happening to our milk-man, the ice-cream man's family and others. He will like that.

As soon as U Nu was out the door Frank said, 'Now we must meet and plan the Mackinac and Caux assemblies.'

. . . The Cross is a positive giving of everything, not an increasing number of self-denials. It means the end of every bit of self-protection, the end of private kingdoms.

It means we stop living inside ourselves, and live out in the world.

I've often been overjoyed when someone has begun to get honest and to have guidance, and failed to move with them to the Cross where they take on their nation and the world as 'this one thing I do' and nothing else.

Thank God for Holland, and particularly one Dutch girl!

April 28th, '59

... You remember when our friend the shipyard worker from Clydeside first met Frank – Frank's question was, 'What are the problems where you come from?' He didn't ask what some of us might have, 'What are your problems?' The man replied, 'Too few have too much and too many have too little.' 'I hate it,' replied Frank, 'it's selfishness in all of us.' And the guy was enlisted for life. Frank was interested in the real problem – and had a bigger and more fundamental answer.

Frank is very interested in the forthcoming assembly in Japan, but at the same time has a burning desire to clean up Tucson. It is the same with Mackinac. He longs for the Island to be cleaned up, as well as for a conference. I suddenly thought of John 3:16 'God so loved the world that He gave . . .' It doesn't say so loved the team, or the answering idea, but the world.

It's one thing for me to be committed to Frank's care, but he himself is committed to giving Tucson a moral leadership. Unless those of us with him take on his fight our care of him is not what we have been fundamentally called to be and do. Because many of us have not taken on this commission we resist every fresh thrust and change of plan because it may interfere with our self-centred activities.

For Frank the Cross was the starting point of his life's work – for many of us it seems to be the ultimate end point of our experience.

Chapter Eight
FREUDENSTADT

WITH BUCHMAN regaining strength after wintering in the warm climate of Arizona, travel plans were made for him to visit his home town in Pennsylvania. It was a trip he greatly enjoyed, and so did those of us who went with him.

(P to A)
May 7th, '59, Dellwood, NY,
We've had a marvellous time so far. A senior business-man and his wife came in yesterday for two magnificent hours . . . although he's still tippling too much. When he asked after you I said you were much better now, having given up drinking! He nearly swallowed his new upper plate . . . . . .

I'm feeling fine and getting some writing done – but I always find it like pulling teeth – hard and painful!

Allentown, May 9th, '59
Phyll Austin came on the phone to say you had created a masterpiece on her costume as the young Mrs Spriggs in *The Crowning Experience* film. . . . all I can say is that God in his great wisdom seems to have apportioned all the talent to one side of the family!

Today we go for one of those famous Dutch lunches after church – then a visit to one of Frank's life-long friends, about 97, then a visit to his parents' graves and back. He's like a little boy in his joy at being in his home with old friends and in the countryside he loves so much.

Allentown Pa, May 15th, '59
Hi, light of my life,
Today the Muhlenberg College Alumni present Frank with the award of merit. . . everyone is staying for lunch,

all the local people, old friends of Frank, have been invited – so we have a duck dinner for about 60!

... It is a crucial moment in the world. We need not just to diagnose and deplore, but to shoulder the lesson and the burden that the diagnosis implies. Frank's greatest failure at the moment would be to neglect to do the planning and thinking for the nations. But for many of us that would not in our minds be our chief sin – it would be not getting on with the wife, or with one of our colleagues ... I'm afraid for a great many their idea is no greater than their own personal experience, and that becomes, nine times out of ten, the only thing they talk about. For many of us our vision does not go beyond the person we are talking to being honest and listening to God ... ...

If we dealt with the chief sin against our nations and the Holy Ghost these minor sins would be dealt with as we went along. But that would end the luxury of talking about ourselves all the time – a terrible fate to contemplate. Some of us would have nothing left!

The summer of 1959 saw a time of tremendous activity, with parallel assemblies continuing through the summer months at Caux and Mackinac, the production of a pamphlet which became the most widely-distributed document MRA has ever produced, and at Mackinac a play entitled *Pickle Hill* – about Buchman's early experiments at Penn State College with the way of life that had so captured me, as a young student. It is a great play, with everything in it – music, humour, real-life stories, the answer to drink and bitterness, and the secret of how to change lives and find a faith.

After spending much of the summer with Annejet at the Mackinac assembly, I and a small party set off to winter with Buchman in Tucson. Yet again Annejet remained at Mackinac, this time preparing for showings of plays in Pittsburgh, at a time when the miners had been on strike.

(P to A)
November 13th, '59, Tucson
Thanks for all your help in getting off. The packing was

beyond anything my bags have so far experienced! . . . we visited Frank's family and friends in Minneapolis, . . . and then boarded the train laden with a basket of fruit-cakes and flowers and got to Kansas City that evening after a great day with the trainmen and dining car men, one of whom lived in Little Rock, had 14 children and knew Daisy Bates. [Mrs L C Bates, who had visited Mackinac, was President of the National Association for the Advancement of Colored People in Arkansas, who had risked her life in 1957 taking a group of black children to a white school every morning. It was over the presence of these black children that violent riots had broken out, which in turn had led in part to the creation of the play *The Crowning Experience.*]

Then on Wednesday we had a magnificent time with the train crew – some of whom had travelled with Frank three years ago. He dressed for supper just so he could see them all – including the three cooks – and the barman who came through specially to see him. We are sending a book to each one of them at his home address, and one may get to Mackinac at the weekend. A passenger, a Texas dentist, who observed all Frank did in the diner came to speak to him in his cabin afterwards. We had a first-rate time with him.

The house here is magnificent, complete with a lawn which it did not have before. The milk-man and egg-man were overjoyed to see us, and the plumber.

Annejet joined us in Tucson for Christmas and in January left for a visit to Holland, to see her family after a stay in North America of three-and-a-half years. The weeks and months in Tucson were, typically of life with Buchman, full of people – both in person and by letter – but also increasingly difficult physically. He was losing his sight, and was mostly confined either to bed or to a wheelchair. But, undeterred and in optimistic spirits, he prepared to cross the Atlantic with around 150 people, to attend the Caux assembly.

We arrived in April, and it was wonderful to meet up with Annejet again there.

We spent the summer in Caux, where there were many

national groups working closely together – Brazilian dock-workers with a play entitled *Men of Brazil*, militant Japanese students with their play *The Tiger*, miners from Germany's Ruhr with their play *Hoffnung* (Hope). Each of these groups was not merely performing in a theatre, but actively seeking to relate and pass on the experiences that had transformed their lives and some of the attitudes of their nations. They were in Switzerland, Paris, London, Milan, Rome. And, though confined to bed much of the time, Buchman's mind worked like that of a man half his age, with more than usual vigour and imagination, thinking and planning for the young men and women with their various productions, relating it all to the world we lived in.

After Christmas at Caux, Buchman took about 30 of us to Italy, for several weeks, before returning to Switzerland again. Annejet was in Holland in the meantime, for the launching of *The Crowning Experience* film, rejoining me at Caux in the spring.

Buchman and I stayed in a Milan hotel. The waiter who brought his meal (which I shared, often with one or two others as well, whoever might be present – we always seemed to have all our needs met from his single order) was a member of the Communist Party. At breakfast Buchman asked me to give him one of our books. I did. At lunch, he asked me to give him some of our magazines. I did.

At supper, he asked me to give him some more. I remonstrated that the man had hardly had time to read what we had already given him. 'That's your trouble – you hold back!' Buchman said. He knew his man – for the waiter was distributing the material Buchman had asked me to give him, not only to the hotel staff and to fellow party-members. That was the point I had missed.

As we waited for the waiter and breakfast the next morning Buchman said, 'My aim is to give Jesus Christ to every man I meet, including this waiter who is about to bring me my food.'

The waiter became his firm friend, and brought along most of the staff to a special showing of our latest film which the manager of the hotel arranged in the ballroom.

One of the things that rejoiced Buchman the most that March was the news of the successful première of the film

94

of *The Crowning Experience* in Rome. He himself devoutly believed in the power of that film to affect people and situations, and was deeply unhappy that certain of his colleagues had decided to give it a less-than-priority rating in their forthcoming programme.

This fact, coming as it did at a time when Buchman was possessed with a feeling of great urgency about the world situation and its need for Moral Re-Armament, led him to instigate a series of daily meetings at Caux for his force. He himself was often not well enough to be present, but had his thoughts conveyed by Howard and others, including myself.

He longed to re-awaken God's perspective, something which he felt was lacking, even though previously he had seen it in them. But perhaps, at long distance and indirectly, the plan misfired, and people became victims of the collective and human desire to find scapegoats, end the discomfort and restore an equilibrium. In any event Buchman's thoughts and messages may well have become elaborated on or edited as they passed from person to person. Any who did manage to speak to Buchman personally and directly found an immediate sense of friendship and affection.

In June 1961, on his birthday, Buchman barely had the strength to prepare and deliver his customary address. It was entitled 'Brave Men Choose'. By late July he was really very weary, and in spite of the fact that two Asian Prime Ministers were expected at the assembly in August – or perhaps because of that fact – he decided to go for a short rest to the Black Forest, to the hotel where he had stayed in the past. Peter Howard remained at Caux, working with others on the daily running of the assembly. Morris Martin and I and one or two others accompanied Buchman to Germany. None of us realised he would never return.

July 30th, '61, Freudenstadt,
Dear Annejet,

Had a nightmare last night – dreamt we had to entertain a US Presidential Candidate to dinner! ... Apart from that it was quite active. Frank was awake every hour. They say that is the effect of the air here in Freudenstadt for the first few days – you are tired but don't feel sleepy, then you get out-of-sorts for two or three days, and wish you'd never come, then you begin to sleep! Well we shall see. I had my out-of-sorts day yesterday. I was short on sleep, Frank was very active, it was raining.

. . . for your information, we shall definitely be here three weeks. The food continues to be out of this world.

One of the things I had recently heard Buchman say lingered in my mind in those days of quiet in the Black Forest. 'Time does not heal past sins – bury the past, and you bury God's power with it. Human nature is not very interesting unless you have victory.'

(P to A)
August 2nd,

. . . .This morning I apologised to a friend for bitterness that had been stored away ever since he spoke to me after that meeting on June 1st! I had covered it with activity but it was there. And quite strong too. I suddenly felt what millions must feel, but who have no answer. I felt my friend was so wrong, and wrongly motivated in what he said – but in the night I felt sincerely how wrong I had been in my feelings towards him. It has been a valuable and at the same time costly experience.

. . . The Governor-General of East Pakistan and the Pakistan Ambassador to Bonn were here for Sunday lunch – a great time.

August 4th,

We've just taken Frank in his chair along Frank Buchmanweg [renamed in 1956 in his honour, the place where he was walking in 1938 when the concept of 'Moral Re-Armament' clarified in his mind as being the world's greatest need at that time] and up for lunch. But it really tired him. He doesn't have much strength. Morris and I are getting some tennis – hallelujah!

At 2 pm on August 6th Buchman had a sharp pain in his chest. The local specialist, Dr Dehler, came immediately and helped ease the pain. During the next hours Buchman slipped into unconsciousness from time to time – but each time he recovered his first thought was to ask for any fresh news that had come in.

There was a further shock on the afternoon of August 7th, and he died at 9.45 that evening. Till the last he was struggling to express what he felt to be a nation-saving truth – 'Why not let Britain be guided by God? Why not let God run the world?'

Chapter Nine

FILLING AN EMPTY PLACE

I ACCOMPANIED Buchman's body, after a farewell service in Germany, to New York and on to Allentown, where he was to be buried. We were flown to New York in a military transport plane on one of its regular trips. I was exhausted and slept for most of the journey.

As I stepped from the car in Allentown I was handed a telegram to say that my Dad, now aged 85, was seriously ill in Swift Current, Saskatchewan.

I took the next available flight to Western Canada, where Annejet joined me from Caux. I missed Buchman's funeral service and burial.

Annejet and I had a week with Dad. He was dying from kidney failure. We were with him on Sunday, August 20th as he left us, so peacefully it was almost like going to sleep, just as the sun was coming up over his beloved prairies. His last words were, 'Bless the Lord, O my soul'.

We took him to Vegreville, where he first came from Britain in 1909. It seemed as if all the countryside came to bid him farewell. Many many old friends came to the service, including Ben Hawkins.

I spoke at the service, from a heart full of gratitude for his companionship, his rugged battle for Truth, his Scots heritage and his rich sense of humour. He had said to us earlier, 'When my time comes, just say Don Campbell has moved up from the cellar to the living room.'

He rests beside my mother and sister, under three pine trees overlooking the prairie.

To lose the two men who had meant most to me so quickly, within two weeks of each other, was a heavy blow. I miss them both: Dad for the home life and companionship he provided, and Buchman who fought in season and out that I grow into the person God had in mind. Such a friend is rare and you sorely miss him when you lose him.

Dad fought for everyone he met to do the will of God. He lived purity – he depended on God and not on people. He had a faith and he spread the spirit of Jesus Christ.

Chief Walking Buffalo, then 90 years of age himself, called me on the telephone when he heard the news of my Dad, and said, 'You have lost your father. I believe in God and he knows what's best for us. I pray God to comfort you. When we die our souls go back to where we came from . . . . . . Have courage, we will fight all the harder.'

Before his death Buchman expressed his vision for the leadership of the work of MRA after he was gone: that it would be led by a cabinet of friends. But at the time of his death there had been too much dependence on him to have his vision immediately realised. At this moment Peter Howard was magnificently used by God.

It was not easy for him. He told me once he believed that leadership has nothing to do with power, and everything to do with service. He was not the only one to believe he had an important rôle to play. But for some that belief was not so much a selfless obedience to the will of God as a self-serving reach for position and power. It is something I knew to be part of my own make-up.

I had the privilege of working closely with Peter Howard in so many parts of the world, and of keeping in constant contact through letters whenever our paths diverged. He had immense energy and an enormous capacity for work.

In September '61, just a few weeks after the deaths of Buchman and my Dad, Peter and Doë, with two of their children, invited Annejet and myself to visit them at Hill Farm, their Suffolk home, and then took us fishing at Ullapool in northern Scotland. It was a very precious time.

After that holiday Annejet and I made our first visit to the island of Canna. To be on the land where Dad was born was a deep satisfaction. It filled an empty place in my life – which up till then I could only imagine. We visited my grandfather's forge, his cottage where my father was born, and met a man who used to tend sheep with Dad when they were both boys.

To meet the people of the island explained a bit more of my Dad's character. He went out in his spirit to everyone he met. He would walk the length of a train to be sure there was not a passenger on board he might know. The people of the island treated my wife and me in the same generous spirit.

Then Annejet and I went to London – where two of Howard's plays, *The Ladder* and *The Hurricane*, were to be performed, and I was to take a part in each. *The Ladder* is a short and deeply moving play, dealing with the ambitions and drive for success as a man climbs his career ladder, and the simplicity of Christ's alternative. *The Hurricane*, a full three-act play, is set in the heart of the freedom struggle of an African country, and starred Muriel Smith in an extraordinarily powerful rle.

Peter Howard made a short trip to the far East, from where he wrote me, including sending me an early, as yet unfinished, script of the play I was due to perform in.

(PDH to Paul)
November 21st '61
Dear Paul,

Thank you so much for your valued letter which awaited me here. If we are right in our belief that Governments now must undertake the task of morally rearming whole peoples, then we must help men who are not saints to do what needs to be done. The moral battle is essential and I am praying to be taken to the depths of peoples' lives each day. But we must decide to end the dirty self-righteousness which uses someone else's weakness to secure our own control of a work that should be God's ... ...

I await the arrival of the suggestions for *The Hurricane* before sending you the rough outline which came to me in Tokyo, and which should reach me, typed, today. I'm thankful to be able to share these things with you. Give me perspective on anything where you see I need it. But I mean to tell you what I feel. Unless we fight all out in honesty we shall miss the challenge of the times.

That year, 1961, Annejet and I spent Christmas at Hill Farm with the Howard family. It was such a change from the

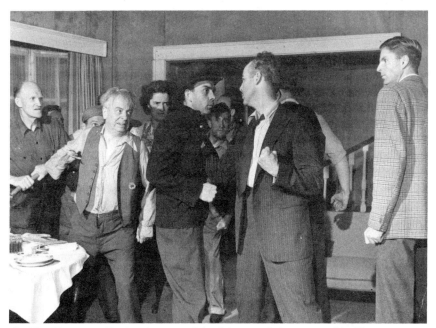

'In *The Forgotten Factor*, the part of the labour agitator seemed to fit my personality.' (with Howard Reynolds)

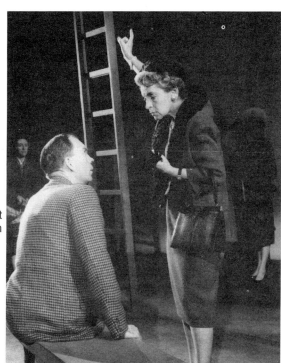

Peter Howard's one-act play, *The Ladder*, with Phyllis Konstam.

previous 19 years that I had spent, closely at Buchman's side, being woken many times in the night, shaping my days to his needs, a certain unavoidable routine. I was grateful for Peter and Doë's heart-warming friendship.

In January Peter took the casts of the plays *The Ladder* and *The Hurricane* on a tour of Britain. Annejet went to Holland, where, by this time, she was expecting our first child. In my wisdom I anticipated it would be a boy, and in my own mind had given the child my father's name.

(P to A)
January 27th, '62, Aberdeen.
A good and uneventful trip, the train arriving on time. Cece [Broadhurst] and I share a room. We need the electric heater constantly – paid for by a shilling at a time!

Look after wee Donald! . . . The peace and power of a mother's heart is all part of it. He will become one of God's great men!

January 23rd, '62 Aberdeen
Last night was a very good house, which immensely pleased the manager. The maid in the hotel serving cocoa in the lounge afterwards said to us, 'Everyone is talking of how wonderful the plays were tonight. I will be in there tomorrow night.'

Many came with real question marks, and went away enthusiastic.

Cece is a good companion – he makes the early morning coffee. It is quite chilly – a good wind from the sea blows through our (closed!) windows.

January 28th, '62, Aberdeen
Last night the manager of the theatre said, 'We thought you would make about £800 here. A good run by a good company makes about £1000. Actually you have taken in £1400.'

The fishwives on the docks here have been marvellous. There were 60 out to see the play on Friday. We have been down to the docks with them, and Muriel Smith had three hours there Thursday morning, singing and speaking with them.

These have been matchless days. As one councilwoman put it, 'You have knocked Aberdeen sideways. We all know you are right. The thing is, have we the courage to do it?'

The wife of a couple in whose home we were for tea yesterday said, 'These are just about the finest professional productions I have ever seen.'

February 4th, '62 Edinburgh

We have had a great week. 5650 people have been to see the plays, including the Provost of Edinburgh, the Provosts of five surrounding towns, 14 of the Edinburgh City Council and many of the leading families. The head of the Industrial Chaplains said, 'It is great. It is brilliant. It is up to the standard of John Bunyan.' The secretary of the Edinburgh Missionary Society said, 'It is the most courageous presentation of the Gospel I have ever seen on the stage. These plays are a must for anyone who is a thinker.'

. . . The fireman in the theatre said, 'I've been with the theatre since 1917, and this is the finest company I have ever worked with.'

. . . My thought is to spend more leisure time with God so I can have more effective time with people.

February 8th, '62, Edinburgh

This morning the Duke of Hamilton personally showed us over Holyrood House. Most impressive. Particularly all the many paintings of Scottish kings which were done by Dutchmen in the 17th century, the best tapestries from Brussels, and some are Flemish, and the woodcarvings and ceilings were done by Dutch brought over by Charles II. I felt very much at home with the Dutch influences!! J. Ruthven [an ancestor of friends of ours] was one of those who climbed the stairs to Mary Queen of Scots' bedchamber to stab her private secretary – an Italian! 13 other noble ruffians joined him, and the body was left with 56 stab-wounds. So I've had quite a morning. . . .

. . . Mr Sing and a Miss Song have been married in South Africa, and a little Sing-Song is expected shortly – at least that is what the BBC says.

February 13th, '62, Brighton

I had quite a rough time on Saturday in Edinburgh, because I had to leave the stage towards the end of *The Hurricane* and just reached the curtain when I brought up my lunch. The audience did not notice anything wrong, so by God's gift we got away with it. Then I went to bed with hot water-bottles for 20 minutes and was able to reappear for the last shows, but with fever. I think it is this pregnancy!

February 16th, '62 Brighton.

The Philips Dictaphone has finally reached me. It is a beautiful instrument. I am delighted with it. It will make so much possible with so little effort. Do tell your Father how much I value it – it is a treasure.

July 15th, '62 Mackinac

I am writing from Petoskey, where this morning I brought a man for an appendectomy. Blanton felt distress yesterday, and his wife consulted me about his condition, as a second opinion. I had a strong feeling I should go to him at 7.00 this morning and found him with acute appendicitis. We had to get him to hospital immediately, which meant we had to get the coast-guard's boat for a 10 mile journey over the water, then a 10 mile ambulance ride. While being examined by the surgeon at the hospital he developed acute pain. I was in the operating theatre with him when he was opened 20 minutes later, and a very badly swollen and ruptured appendix was discovered. The surgeon believes the sudden pain was the rupturing. The miracle of God's timing was literally life-saving. As it is, Blant will be a minimum of two weeks in this hospital. . . .

A very good time with Phil last night. He is deeply run by ambition which keeps his work just one long exhausting frustration and effort and despondency over the size of the problem. A lot of people try to do God's will and work without God – which may perhaps be the height of ambition!

July 17th, '62 Mackinac

Blant is doing well, uncomfortable as would be expected, but feeling a lot better than he did 24 hours ago . . . . . . Yesterday I had an excellent letter from Frank Sladen and his wife, reminiscing on the past and saying how MRA had brought them both to a more realistic relationship with Christ. Plus a cheque. I was very touched by their thought. It was [Peter Howard's book] *Frank Buchman's Secret* that had moved them so much.

When Buchman died I knew it was the end of one period in my life. The knowledge that from this time forward I would have much more freedom brought a certain feeling of relief and a desire to be once more in control of my life. But I made the error of thinking that a commitment of my life could be totally or partly withdrawn. In my eagerness to forge my own way, I stopped drawing on the Almighty's resources for everything that I needed. I depended on my own will and efforts. Ultimately of course I was neither happy, nor at peace, and I must have made life hard at times for those around me.

(P to A)
July 25th, '62, Mackinac

I have had very illuminating days here. God has marvellously provided the place and setting where certain truth could get through. Mackinac represents 20 years of association with Frank . . . Over the last days I have realised that I worked for 20 years with a man who put God first, but I often put Frank first. I have never before accepted the full truth of it. Frank tried time and again to break me of it . . .

. . . I marvel with intense wonder at the love of God which has never let me go. It is beyond human understanding, but it is true. It is of course the very heart of the struggle in the world – men enslaved to men, or the free servants of the living God. I was able to talk about it at lunch yesterday with eight of my closest friends and colleagues. I do not want to project my sin on anyone else but I believe this may affect every one of us who worked with Frank.

A work or a movement – even one with the highest of callings – can become a medium for the expression of unchanged human ambitions, for a sense of worthwhileness, achievement, power. A person can become a source of security, judgement, guidance, attitudes. Both the movement and the person, good in themselves, become destructive because they are made idols and take the place God alone should have in our lives.

I realised that I had put Buchman on a pedestal, uncritically highlighting to others his gifts of spiritual leadership. I did once or twice venture to correct him, when I felt he'd made a mistake, and he was a man who was grateful for that kind of friendship. But by and large I was happy to reflect what seemed glorious about him, and to bask in it. For being with Buchman was success, and it fed my ambition. It made me heady and high – above 'lesser mortals'. Thank God Frank's was such a good life – purposeful and creative. Nevertheless he was just a man, and would never have wanted to be a substitute for Christ in my life or anyone else's.

I am sure it was in his passionate loyalty to Christ's answer in the hearts of men and women that he saw his work winning the future.

(P to A)
July 31st, '62, Mackinac
Your letter from Arnhem arrived yesterday. We had spent a good part of the day in Petoskey seeing Blanton who should be out later this week. Yesterday I sent Jane to Ann Arbor because of her neck, it looks like an acute disc. I was up to 1.30 am with Keith, the night before last, with an acute gastric ulcer. I seem to be developing a medical practice!

I once asked a friend with an ulcer if he were harbouring a resentment against someone. I explained that, medically, if I were to put a gastroscope into his stomach, the lining would appear all reddened, like the face of an angry man.

He denied that he had any resentment in his life. Next day he came back to tell me that actually the relationship between him and his father was not right. He went to see his father to straighten out what he could, from his side. He had no further recurrence of his abdominal pain.

(P to A)
August 3rd, '62, Mackinac
. . . . It was just a year ago today I helped take Frank on that last wheelchair ride on Frank Buchmanweg.

August 8th, '62, Mackinac
These have been 40 hours of the greatest significance for America. Bill Keeler, the oil man, who is part Chero-kee-Indian, together with other senior industrialists, was welcomed by Chief Walking Buffalo, Chief David Crow-child and Princess Fisher who represents the 60 American tribes in Washington. We had pitched the big teepee from Alberta on the lawn approaching the theatre.

Keeler said of Walking Buffalo, 'My people once had character. It is gone. But some still have it and the Chief has maintained that strength.' He was very moved by it. The film-studio here bowled these men over.

They saw the African film, *Freedom*, that afternoon, then on stage *The Real News*, and after dinner we stayed in the dining room and had music and talk. Then after the 7.30 am meeting yesterday they had *El Condor* as a play and the Latin Americans spoke. After lunch they had the film of *Men of Brazil*, then a session with them over tea, then a performance of *The Ladder*, and after dinner *The Dictator's Slippers* on stage. And after that a recep-tion.

It's been non-stop but glorious. Blant was able to be up for the first lunch and yesterday for the tea and even-ing. Keeler said as he left, 'You will now see the pace in the oil industry pick up.' He sees in MRA the instrument for bringing to birth a God-controlled world. Those were his own words.

Chapter Ten

FATHERHOOD AT 50

OUR FIRST DAUGHTER was born on 22nd September, 1962 in Holland. Annejet's parents had generously invited us to come and live with them, as we did not have a home of our own at that point.

In Holland, most babies are born at home, if all seems to be going well during pregnancy. A very dear friend and competent nurse, Tjits Hoekstra, came to help. Annejet woke up at five that morning and said to me, 'I think something is happening.' I rushed downstairs to call the doctor, but I must have dialled it wrongly in my nervous excitement, because I got some irate Dutchman on the other end of the phone, who was not exactly pleased to be wakened at that hour.

Finally the baby arrived at 11.30 at night, a daughter. What a joyous miracle it was. Annejet's whole family had just returned from a wedding, and stood around the bed in their finery admiring the new arrival.

We called her after my sister and my mother – Edith Anne.

It is not every man who becomes a father for the first time at 50 – with the attendant joys of getting up at strange times in the night, only this time to a rather more strenuous call than I had experienced in my earlier medical career. There is a lot to learn, in the art of fatherhood. I can still picture Edith Anne under the Christmas tree at her grandparents' home, aged about three months, with the candlelight sparkling in her eyes.

A couple of months later I was far afield again, this time in Japan. *Space Is So Startling*, a musical by Peter Howard based on the super-power space-race, was invited with its large cast and company to Japan for two months in 1962. Annejet, in Holland with Edith Anne, was again the recipient of various letters from me. I wrote as often as I could.

(P to A)
November 23rd, '62, Osaka,

Yesterday was a big day. We were with the Junior Chamber of Commerce in Kobe for two hours, a turkey Thanksgiving at our hotel with senior pressmen and others.

. . . Many need the truth of the story of the Good Samaritan who did what was needed for fallen, cheated and wounded humanity while everyone else went by on the other side, so proud of their good moral living or standards.

We got to Tokyo on Sunday, put on *Space* in Yokohama this coming week, have the Odawara assembly December 1st-8th, put on *Space* December 10th, 11th, 12th, in Tokyo and leave for London ready to mount *Space* in the Westminster about December 19th. Today is a holiday!

November 29th, '62, Tokyo

We had a geisha party with, among others, the President of Nippon University. There were eight of us, eight girls or more, sake, beer and a colossal meal. We ploughed through. The owner of the place is unscrupulous and fat, but shrewd. He began to get the point. The girls were fascinated, and the President wants the play for his university. . . . . You must be frozen in. I have had no letter since Saturday – not complaining, mind you, just presenting the facts!

December 4th, '62, Odawara

Your letter of 27th came last evening. Roses and white flowers adorn my room today – put there by Mrs Kubyawa who arranged the flowers at our wedding, and who remembered your yen for red roses!

I don't see any reason why your friends in Holland shouldn't do *The Ladder* (Peter Howard's one-act play) commercially. . . . Professionalism is not only getting paid for a high skill, it is giving the maximum every second, no matter how you feel. A professional actor is not run by feelings while on the stage, and a life-changer is not run by feelings on the stage or off the stage. But I whole-heartedly agree – it must be super theatre. If not, it's not MRA.

December 8th, '62, Tokyo

Masa (Shibusawa) and I went yesterday for an hour with the President of the Mitsui Mining Co. He is the one who takes the tough attitude to labour. So I began by saying I felt Japanese management was not tough enough with labour – not tough enough to out-revolutionise and change them. Anyone can smash the other man, and remain soft, comfortable and selfish. But to change the other man and unite a nation takes a lot more toughness. He said 'MRA is a much bigger idea, and better, than I had understood.'

Then we had over an hour with the head of the Miners' Union nationally. They are calling a national strike next week, so he was up to his neck in negotiations and strategy. We had lunch with him. His first question was, 'What do you think of our struggle?' I replied, 'It has got to be won, and I want to see the miners, the industry and the nation and the world benefit by the solution.' At one point he said, 'How many members do you have in Japan?' I replied, '90 million.' It gave him an absolutely fresh conception. I said, 'I am convinced if you and management and government think of building a new world, you will reach the right solution on this crisis by considering what is right and not who is right on every problem.'

I told him MRA is not a personal improvement society, run by a few to oppose Communism. He laughed, and said, 'That of course is the way we in labour have been thinking.' He left us promptly at 1 pm to go to a strike strategy meeting.

December 11th '62, Tokyo

Peter (Howard) and I had lunch with the head of the Atomic Energy Commission. He was earlier in jail under the Americans, whom he cordially hates. He developed the first TV station. His paper circulates seven million copies a day. He is now on a programme to abolish golf widows (you will be glad to hear!) by having a children's playground and entertainment for wives of golfers next door. Then we saw colour TV for the first time.

Koga, the head of the National Mineworkers, with whom I had lunch, spent one-third of his time that evening talking of MRA to the labour men of the Mitsui Mining Co. They reported the fact to the President, whom we had seen that morning.

And, just to prove that the traffic was not all one-way, some months after Edith Anne was born, Annejet went away for a short holiday to Switzerland, leaving me to look after our daughter.

(P to A)
February 1st, '63, Wassenaar

. . . EA is pushing down macaroni and cheese. She even tried to eat the casserole dish. She continues very cheerful, and just about rolls herself over on the bed. You had better get your muscles in good trim to keep up with her when you get back!

. . . the helplessness I feel in front of the child. As parents we can do everything for her except the one thing that really matters. That God alone can do. But I need to be aware of that need and that powerlessness as I enjoy her and love her for what she is. We must never lose sight of what real love for the child involves.

Annejet and I went on a six-week assignment that spring, with Peter and Doë Howard, and two intrepid senior ladies – Dame Flora Macleod, Chief of the Clan Macleod in Scotland, and Mrs Charlotte van Beuningen, in whose home we were now living in Holland. It was a rare privilege to travel with them, through Japan, Hong Kong and India. Tjits Hoekstra offered to look after Edith Anne while we were away, and we gratefully accepted.

In June I was back in England for a short stay.

111

(P to A)
June 19th, '63, Hill Farm

Yesterday afternoon I came here to stay with Peter and Doë for a couple of nights. This morning we got a message off to America, asking when they want *Space Is So Startling* . . . I think more deeply engrained in me than I realise is the belief that to seek others' advice and opinion is a sign of weakness. A grudging listening to others means a grudging listening to God. I have had a fierce resolve to be independent. I will be most grateful for any illumination you have for me on this point or any others.

June 27th, '63, London

I was most grateful for your thought on the ambitious motives which have played a part in keeping our plans indefinite. There is a drive to measure up in men's eyes which robs me of God and God of me. It keeps me from being myself in God's hands, for his purposes.

I did go to the United States that autumn, and Annejet joined me for Christmas in Los Angeles. And early the next year we moved our family base to Canada, where we had been generously invited by John and Clare Hallward to share their home in Ottawa. It was a busy time in Eastern Canada, with showings of the revolutionary Latin American play, *El Condor*, written and acted by students whose lives had been changed by their contact with MRA. Led by General Hugo Bethlem of Brazil, they gave performances in Québec which led to many introductions to the leadership of all aspects of the life of the Province, and they travelled widely across the rest of Canada.

In the summer of 1964, Mackinac Island was the focus of the largest youth conferences it had ever seen, with 2,000 delegates. There were two main conference sessions, from June through to August, and it was a hive of the best creative energy that the American continent has to offer. Plays were produced and filmed by the young conference delegates, in the excellently-equipped film studios, and a new musical revue came to birth. It started life as a 'Showboat', giving performances of songs and sketches on an old supply barge travelling around Lake Michigan. It developed by the following year into a full and superb stage presentation – *Sing-Out*.

It was a glorious creation – with all the colour and humour, music and harmony that North America has to offer. In its cast were young people from all over the continent, from West to East and North to South, including representatives of the Native American peoples of Canada and New Mexico, of whom there had been over 200 at the conference. The aim of the show was to mobilize the energy and imagination of young people of every race, class and creed behind a patriotic determination to build a nation that could lead the whole world forward.

During the conference sessions, the delegates listened attentively to many distinguished speakers – including Chief Walking Buffalo, senior political figures, sportsmen and also Peter Howard. Such was the interest shown by what Howard had to say that he was invited after the conference to university campuses all over the continent, to give his uncompromising vision for what the young people of America could be and do.

Opening the conference, he had said, 'The whole world stands or falls on America. If America fails, the world fails. America will not fail. America morally re-armed will capture the allegiance of the entire world.'

The conference day began at 6.15 am, with calisthenics, and continued through the main morning plenary session, and into workshops in drama, television, journalism, radio, cooking, seminars on current world problems; mandatory sports programmes in the afternoon, evening programmes which were very often theatrical or musical, and curfew at 10.30 pm. After the three week conference was over, the delegates went back to their home areas, in many cases taking with them guests from other parts of the continent, or from Asia, Africa, Latin America and Europe who had attended the conference. A group of about 30 drove across Canada, meeting the mayors and Members of the Legislatures in each town they passed through, speaking on radio and TV, giving their convictions and hopes and decisions for the future.

Some weeks later, I found myself in Japan, at the time of the Tokyo Olympics, meeting again with some of the men and women whom I knew from earlier visits. Annejet remained in Ottawa with Edith Anne. During this time Peter Howard was criss-crossing the North American continent, with countless speaking engagements in colleges, and on television, meeting students, military and political leaders and the press.

(P to A)
October 27th, '64, Tokyo
    ... Peter comes over on the 11th and I need to see him on arrival. I had some further thoughts following the letter he sent me. Frank was like a father and also the founder of the work. I regarded it as an honour to be with him, and it also bolstered my pride. But those of us he trained are much the same age group – and being put in the position of needing to learn from Peter and others suddenly brings out all the pride which has always been there ... God resists the proud – because the proud resist him. I have tried to make what I was doing as important as what anyone else was doing. It is so silly – self-centred and godless ... Thank God we grow.

(PDH to Paul)
October 25th, '64, London
Dear Paulus,
    ... I was moved by what you wrote to me about my being 'in charge' and the other matters. My life is not my own. It belongs to God and this fellowship of ours. Nor do I one whit feel more 'in charge' than you – or anyone else who will bear the brunt with us. It is simply that, for good or ill, in the modern world somebody has to wear the label of final responsibility, for otherwise men think there is no responsibility and indeed an irresponsibility that they can ignore or destroy. My faith is that if we stick together and live always in the daylight, God will give us all we need.

In January 1965 Annejet and I – leaving Edith Anne in the care of Tjits Hoekstra in Ottawa – went to Brazil, to participate with Peter and Doë Howard, Rajmohan Gandhi of India, grandson of the Mahatma, and many others in a venture which Peter felt at the time to be one of the biggest he had ever undertaken.

The receptions by the political leadership, the Foreign Office, the ordinary people of the shanty-towns, the dock-workers, was unprecedented. Many doors were flung open, and when the Howards moved on to take up invitations from Argentina, Uruguay, Chile and Peru, most of us stayed on in Brazil, continuing what had been begun.

Peter contracted virus pneumonia, and died after only two days in hospital, in Lima, Peru. The news reached us by telex in Recife.

We were numbed and could hardly believe it. I knew I had lost the truest friend I've ever had. I felt definitely handicapped.

A short time later a letter reached me from Peter, written two days before he died:

(PDH to Paul)
23rd February 1965, Lima, Peru
   What is it, Paul, that so often makes you get so high? Is it some small compromise about which you have not been honest? Or is it that you do not realise the way ambition in its drive and falseness takes you over when you leave the Cross? Do think about it because the chance we have is so great and our humble unanimity is the key.
   P.S. Is it just rivalry with me that you have never faced? If so, forgive me if in any way I have made it harder for you. It's the very last thing I wish to do.

This letter shook me deeply. It touched me that he took the time to write when he was in the middle of much activity and already feeling ill. I felt deeply ashamed, and wished I could have talked it all over with him.

After Peter's funeral in Suffolk, Annejet returned to Canada, to be with Edith Anne in Ottawa. I stayed on in Britain.

(P to A)
March 25th, '65, London
   . . . I have always thought I had been such a gift to

everybody – first with my medicine and Buchman, and then the plays. Actually I have been a considerable headache . . .

But then I wrote this in my notebook this morning. 'You are saved by My love and nothing else. You have nothing to bring and nothing you can do. My love and power are massive enough to deal with even you. You do not acknowledge Me by carrying a burden but by accepting Me and My grace. Do not seek transformation, seek Me.' . . .

. . . While Buchman was alive, most of our force were orientated toward him. Then we had Peter. Now there is no single personality of outstanding ability. It must mean we need to reconstruct our relationships with each other through honesty and with God, with a new degree of faith.

April 15th, '65, London

It is so easy to use diagnosis not as a doorway to cure but as an excuse for withdrawal from the sacrifice necessary to help others Godwards. . . . I have at times been committed to my own advancement, like the type of doctor who may try to cure people, but uses their illness to develop his own career.

We are about to have the first opportunity since Peter's death to confer with some of the European force. . . . I have seen the first cut of *Mr Brown Comes Down the Hill* on film. (Peter Howard's powerful play about what might happen if Christ appeared on earth in the latter part of the 20th Century). It is absolutely superb. I have never been so deeply moved by any film.

April 21st, '65, London

You have been a brick in the way you have put up with so much. I am often facile and shallow, with the quip and quick excuse in conversation, which is sometimes funny but always self-centred and shallow. 'Be true to yourself and you cannot be false to any man.'

You have courage and tenacity and a heart, but if your peace and satisfaction of heart is going to depend upon what I or anyone else gives, then you are going to be always unsatisfied. The only way to live with a satisfied heart I know of is to live every moment and do everything with a conscious effort to please Him. I find it immediately translates into giving my best, however I feel, and whatever is going on. It makes God the centre of living, and cuts more quickly at man-pleasing and self-concern, demand and negative thinking than anything else I know.

God loves you the way you love Edith Anne, only more perfectly. He does not hold a grudge against us for the past. He loves the humble and the contrite heart of the child who says sorry, and then goes on never doubting the care and affection of its parents . . . . . .

May 6th, '65, London
. . . What a clutch on my heart your daughter has. The pull of home has been a deep strong tide in my life – so quiet and powerful.

June 29th '65, London
. . . It was a marvellous gift to hear you both on the phone. It will be such fun to be together again. Bringing up children is a new experience, an uncharted sea.

In July, Annejet and Edith Anne returned to London from Canada, and we made our home in one of the big houses in central London, given for the work of Moral Re-Armament after the war. It was to be our family base for the next two years and we were grateful for the fellowship of those we lived with. It was not always easy for any of us, living in a house with 22 other people, but we had a lot of fun. We certainly learned a great deal, and look back on the comradeship of that time with gratitude.

In October 1965, I travelled to the Nordic countries, to fulfil speaking engagements in medical faculties of various universities – something very close to my heart.

(P to A)
October 5th, Copenhagen.
8th wedding anniversary
. . . These have been eight wonderful years, full of

colour and light and shade, action, the unexpected, the unusual, the pain and intense joy of Christ's battle. What the future holds only the Almighty knows, but it is a vast treasure house of inexhaustible riches. To share life with you is a privilege beyond price. I love you with all my heart, and I am grateful beyond my ability to express for all you bring to our marriage, and the best is still to be realised.

The students' club here is 140 years in existence. They have had everyone from Churchill to Kruschev, and at one point invited Goebbels, only to be told by the Foreign Minister that they had to disinvite him. There were about 150 last night, with questions till 10 o'clock . . . One thing is clear, MRA is the most lively of any issue in these countries. It is the only thing that cuts across the painting-the-cabin-while-the-ship-goes-down mentality.

A most valuable dinner in Stockholm with leading doctors and their wives, and a very good time at lunch with the Chief of Police and young student conservative leaders. The Chief says he has often had to deal with youth with an idea, communist or fascist, etc. But today most of the youth he deals with have no ideas – they are empty. He has asked me to reserve time for him the next time I am in Stockholm.

In Uppsala, after I had spoken to a group of medical students, the President of the student body who thanked me said, 'Before Dr Campbell spoke, I was confused about MRA. Now I am still confused, but on a higher level!'

Together with other colleagues from around Europe, I went to Germany in June 1966, to help – as I thought – with preparations and arrangements for a visit from the American *Sing-Out* cast. It was an eye-opener. For reasons I could not understand, many of us were excluded and ignored to the point of discourtesy by our friends who were organising the *Sing-Out* visit. We were angry and puzzled. It seemed as if we were not welcome, except on their terms.

Events over the next year or two confirmed that many of our American friends were determined to go their separate way. *Sing-Out* had begun as a matchless and inspiring

118

musical at Mackinac, aimed at enlisting the youth of America in the world dimension of Moral Re-Armament. But over time the moral and spiritual content of the show was replaced with a more specifically educational and patriotic message. It appeared that the success of the show became more and more the focal point.

Thousands of young people were captivated by the dynamism and spirit of the show. Local *Sing-Out* groups sprang up all over the country. In 1967 it was retitled *Up With People* and separately incorporated the next year under that name. By that time the young people were no longer being exposed to the challenges and demands of obedience to God and his absolute moral standards. After the encounters in Germany, I attempted, with others, to express my unease about it to the people concerned. But some of us in Britain were judgemental and self-righteous about the direction our friends in North America and elsewhere took. We were guilty of taking sides and of cutting people off, publicly and privately, if they had links with *Up With People*. We accused old friends of betrayal. Our attitudes only widened the gap and strengthened the divisions.

Chapter Eleven

THE GOAT BECAME A STILL

IN JULY, 1966, I visited Kenya and India, but was back in London for the birth of our second daughter on October 13th.

She came two weeks early and has been surprising us ever since. Her arrival was evidently imminent at 7.15 in the morning, and we just had time to throw a few things for Annejet in a suitcase, get a taxi, and the baby was born at 9.20 am.

The doctor got stuck in the London rush-hour traffic, so the midwife and I delivered the baby – a perfectly formed little girl, with dark hair and dark eyes. We called her Digna, after Annejet's grandmother and eldest sister.

We felt blessed beyond measure, with two daughters! Edith Anne was thrilled with her little sister, and was old enough at four to 'help' look after her.

When Digna was five months old we had some very anxious hours. For a couple of days she had not been eating, vomiting at first but then just lying very quiet, not even crying. It was very eerie. We discovered gall-bladder material on her pillow one morning, and when the doctor came he advised us to rush her to Great Ormond Street Childrens' Hospital.

They operated at once, and found she had had an intusseception, where the bowel becomes obstructed by itself. The swift operation saved her life.

Annejet and I sat in a nearby café, during the operation, wondering what was going to happen. We both had the strong sense that she was not just our child, she belonged to God and he knew what was best for her. All we could do was wait, pray and trust.

She came through the operation triumphantly, and we left her in the care of the nurses – a tiny little thing in an enormous bed, with a wound across her tum, and tubes coming out of her. In fact it was strangely reassuring to see the nurse who looked after her in the hospital, holding the little girl under a tap instead of washing her bottom with a cloth on the bed. She handled her almost like a bit of beef.

When we returned home to Edith Anne the house was so quiet, without the baby . . . But she had made it, and we were grateful beyond words that she had been entrusted to us a second time.

The business of bringing up children was, of course, as new to us as it is to all parents. We wanted them to regard their own touch with God as something very precious. We didn't force them to do the things we believed to be right for them, but we did sit down with them and try to listen to God together when there was something of specific interest to them — for instance a family coming to have tea with us. A child's thought-life is so limited that if you attempt to make your children listen to God regularly each day, all they will probably come up with is, 'I must be nice to my sister and help Mummy with the dishes.' Nothing wrong with that, once in a while, but not every day of their lives!

Of course we made mistakes, a lot of them. But the knowledge that you can listen to God, and not just pray to him, has been a great reassurance.

One of the girls as a small child used to bite her nails and suck her thumb — a cause of irritation to her and to us, but one which she seemed incapable of doing anything about. We together devised a simple method — we tied a bandage round her thumb, and if the bandage was still there the next morning she would get a small coin. It worked — in two weeks it was gone, no more problem.

When she got upset she would lie on the floor, kick her heels and scream. Someone said to us bluntly, 'This child is controlling your lives, and it is as bad for her as it is for you. What will you do about it?'

Annejet and I had a time of quiet and prayer about it, and realising that we couldn't pick up on every single point that we felt was wrong, we decided to insist on certain disciplines which were irrevocable — tidying up the bedroom in the morning, eating up what was on her plate or there would be no dessert, that she shouldn't change her clothes all day long

– and lastly not to be afraid to say 'no' to her when we had to. She was about four. We explained to her that we had decided that this was how it was going to be, and what we expected of her . . . She listened very quietly, said nothing, and the next morning her bedroom was in a terrible mess.

Annejet said to her, 'Well, why don't you tidy up quickly and I'll go and get breakfast ready.' In about half a minute the child appeared downstairs, and when asked if her room was tidy she replied, 'Yes, but don't go and look at it just now!'

We found when we insisted on these simple points that she became a much happier person. Children like to know where they stand, but parents don't always realise it.

In 1967 the leasehold on the big house in central London where we had lived for two years came to an end. It meant 22 of us had to find new accommodation. Annejet's father very generously offered to buy a house for us which would be MRA property. We found the perfect family home in Dulwich, five miles south of central London, near good schools and a big park.

Just before Christmas we moved to our new home. As it is big enough to house two families, we invited the Dodds family to share the home with us. Dickie is a well-known English cricketer, and his and Ann's son, Michael, is just a few months younger than Edith Anne. It was a happy partnership which lasted almost 20 years, and one for which we have been profoundly grateful.

I greatly enjoyed all the games with the girls, as well as cricket and tennis in the garden, and going swimming.

Edith Anne always had a great passion for drama and often wrote plays for the children to perform for us. We watched a variety of productions over the years, including a circus and acrobatics, and countless playlets at Christmastime.

Digna was rather reluctantly dragged into these, and one December day when Edith Anne suggested they again do a play for Christmas Digna pleaded, 'Couldn't we have one Christmas off?' Edith Anne also wrote plays at other times of the year and I was given a great part once, playing a dead body under a blanket.

At school when she was about 13 she had to write an essay about a famous person and produced a 25-page document on Marie Curie. Then she changed it to a play which was performed in our home. She, of course, had the lead rôle, and there were 22 scene changes. It was done with great imagination and improvisation, and we were moved to tears in the scene where Marie died.

The children loved going to the summer conferences at Caux with us, because they were allowed to help, for instance, in the baking kitchen, preparing cakes and cookies for the conference. Digna one summer invited herself to every birthday party that was on, because she knew who was having a cake and when. Edith Anne was allowed to help as receptionist in the small infirmary there, wearing a nurse's uniform of which she was very proud.

(P to A)
January 9th, '68, Caux

I believe that the children are in our custody – but are not our possession. On my knees I turned them over to God absolutely. The next morning my waking thought was, 'I put them in your charge'. It may well be the secret of parenthood. To be responsible but not possessive.

You have a wonderful title for your speech. What I want for my children? Some of the things are – children who stand alone with God, something we arrive at by seeking not father's will or mother's will, or even the childrens' will, but God's will. A concern for the whole world – this alone God can give, but it needs to be practical. A concern to lift the misery of the human condition and the pain in the human heart. Children who are honest, and who learn that because we are honest with them.

During the previous months a new conference and training centre, Asia Plateau, had been built in the hills above Pune, at Panchgani in Western India. The land had been given to Rajmohan Gandhi expressly for this purpose. High in the ghats, it has a wonderful situation, with breath-taking views across the valleys. I was invited to be present at the official opening early in 1968 – a vivid and colourful experience.

(P to A)
January 21st, '68, Panchgani

At least 4000 people came from Panchgani and neighbouring towns and villages, some walking more than 10 miles each way. They stayed most of the day, as did the press which was here in full force. Good stories and pictures today. We have people here from the Philippines, Sri Lanka, Australia, Irène Laure from France, others just in from a visit to Pakistan, and of course from every corner of India itself.

Many miracles happened in those days . . . not my interpretation of events, but that of the people concerned. For instance, two farmers came to Asia Plateau, brothers from a nearby village. They had not spoken to each other for years, such was the bitterness and mistrust between them. It was a feud which had split their small village. After a meeting, during which everyone present was offered the chance to spend a few moments in silence, listening to the inner voice in their hearts, one farmer apologised to his brother, publicly. His brother's response was, 'I've seen many organisations, but here I have found true brotherhood. You have the answer to the divisions destroying the countries. I have experienced a miracle – my brother and I have got together. This is what the country needs. If we are not open to these ideas, then we are traitors to the nation.'

The one who apologised explained why he had done it.

'I was a man with a light-bulb fully wired, but it didn't work. Then a man from Asia Plateau put in the fuse, jiggled the bulb a few times, and suddenly it came alight. I apologised to my brother. We never physically beat each other, but it was a constant tug-of-war.' The two farmers said, 'Let no-one discourage you. We will give our village the inspiration we saw today. Now we have real strength.'

Another story worth recalling is that of the man who was known as the king of the underworld in the area surrounding Panchgani. He had 200 men selling illicit liquor. For seven days a leader of one group of workers in the town had tried to get this influential man, Bhil, to visit Asia Plateau. And every day for eight days he was told by the man's wife, 'he is not at home'.

It was well-known that Bhil started his day's drinking at 9.00 am, becoming abusive and often incoherent by lunchtime, so the workers' leader turned up at his home on the morning of the eighth day at 7.00 am. Bhil sent out a message – 'Don't bother me'. The workers' leader went to the temple and prayed, 'I have been after this man for over a week, so make him listen now.'

He returned to the back door of the house, and asked the wife to stop Bhil from drinking that morning. He found something to occupy the cronies who usually drank with Bhil, and sent them off. Then, from early in the morning until 4.00 pm this workers' leader never left the home of Bhil – he had no lunch, not even a cup of tea.

He had enlisted the help of the local doctor and his car to bring Bhil to Asia Plateau. The car was parked by the front door, and finally Bhil yielded and went. He no sooner arrived than he sent for the head man of the neighbouring village, a close confidant. It was said that these two men used to supply goat's milk for Gandhiji, but in the fullness of time the goat had turned into a still. Bhil was much won when Rajmohan Gandhi said he believed the worst rascal was he who thought he was a saint; and he himself had been that kind of rascal. The man who knows he is a rascal and gets honest can walk close with God.

Next morning Bhil astonished everyone by sending a man at 6.30 am to the workers' leader who had originally brought him to Asia Plateau, getting him out of bed and asking him to come to the market place to meet Bhil. So there they were, at 7.00 am in the morning in the market place, planning how to raise money to support the ongoing building programme of Asia Plateau.

About ten days before all this happened there had been evidence of vigorous opposition to the work of MRA in Panchgani, but after the change which took place in Bhil one of those most vociferous in protest approached this same workers' leader and said, 'I want you to forget all that has happened, and all that has been said. Keep your heart clean. I did not realise you were working for such a great thing. Let us now forget the past and work for the future. Come and meet with us tomorrow, and help us plan for our next meeting with Rajmohan Gandhi and his friends.'

(P to A)
March 30th '68, Panchgani

... Tomorrow we have a big meeting in the village called by the man who drank 2500 rupees worth of liquor a year. He is a miracle and came this morning to plan the afternoon.

Tell EA: This morning I went to the Asia Plateau school for the children of the people who work here. The children all sit on the ground. They had all seen your picture and Digna's and are very thankful for the clothes you sent. I had a map of the world, and I showed them all the places in Europe, and Africa, and Australia, and Asia, and America and Canada where I have been sending the news of how they have stopped lying and stealing and have begun to help their mothers in the house, and to build a school, and in this way they are helping to change the world.

Then we all were quiet together. They were all given a cup of milk, although some didn't have cups, they just had tins. I gave them five simple rules I have learned about life – don't steal from one another; don't cheat one another; don't tell lies to one another; don't carry hate in your heart for anyone and love everybody else the way you love yourself. I had tears in my eyes when I left them. They have so little to wear and to eat and yet they are so content when they do what God tells them in their hearts to do – really wonderful children. When I went to school at your age, I once stole some coloured chalk, and when I got home I put colour all over the side of a wooden shed. Oh my! Everybody could see it, and wanted to know where I got the chalk. I lied about it and said I found it, but my Mother and Daddy and teacher knew better, so I took it back, and I think I got a good spanking.

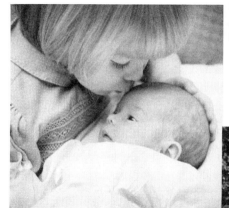

'Edith Anne, at four, was old enough to "help" look after Digna.'

'We found the perfect family home in Dulwich.'

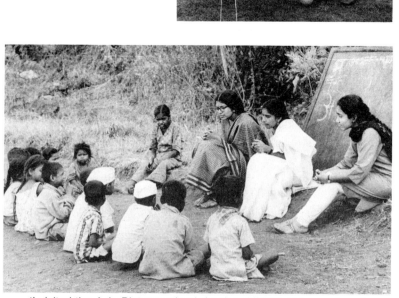

'I visited the Asia Plateau school, for the children of the workers.'

Chapter Twelve
AN EYE-OPENER

IN JANUARY 1970 Annejet and I returned to Canada, to attend the wedding of the Marquis of Graham, of Scotland, and Cathy Young of Ottawa, niece of Lester Pearson, the former Prime Minister. Seumas Graham, a good friend of ours, had played the bagpipes both at our wedding and on the occasion when we announced our engagement, and we had worked together in many parts of the world.

It was wonderful to be back in Canada after five years. We were welcomed with open arms by Ted and Audrey Porter and were their guests in Montréal.

It was in the course of that short visit of about a month that I began to understand the extent of the isolation and separation felt by many of my old friends in Canada and the United States at that time. In effect there was a gulf, a division in the work of Moral Re-Armament on the two sides of the Atlantic, caused in part by the separate developments of thought, understanding and action during the previous few years.

Letters had been sent across the ocean, often judging and blaming. Accusations were made which still today are keeping some of the divisions going. When someone wants to believe right is on his side, it is not hard to tailor information about the people he is criticising to sharpen his argument when he conveys it to his friends. Perhaps, for various reasons, there was a climate of thought that was only too ready to believe the worst about people.

Looking back on it all, I think many of us living and working in Britain withdrew too quickly, in self-righteous judgement, instead of more of us going over to North America and putting all our cards on the table and humbly seeking a way forward together. There were many places where we ourselves were wrong. Maybe some felt that their chance for leadership had now come, and they were going to make the most of it. I know that thought certainly crossed my mind at one point. I am an ambitious man – not something of which I am proud. But could it be that a humble acknowledgement of my ambition might have helped others find freedom from controlling motives in their own lives? A fresh and undemanding honesty might have untangled some of the many threads that had contributed to such a sorry tapestry. If so, it was something I missed, and which I deeply regret.

In Europe we had tried to continue the work of MRA as we understood it, after the deaths of Buchman and Howard. Plays by Howard and others were staged at the Westminster Theatre in London, for example, reaching people in industry, civic life, education, politics and the diplomatic world.

In some ways people countered the 'liberalisation' of *Up With People* with something of a fortress mentality in Britain, in an attempt to preserve the original qualities of MRA.

Possibly that approach swung the pendulum too far in the opposite direction, so that unwritten rules and regulations took great prominence, and people felt strait-jacketed.

And then came the day when a handful of men and women in North America decided before God that they would relaunch the work of Moral Re-Armament, as conceived by Buchman, in Canada and the United States. In legal terms, this involved a court case over the use of the name, 'Moral Re-Armament', and the resources which had been given, often sacrificially, and always in good faith, to further the work of MRA over the years.

A miracle of healing began in the USA when five of those trying to carry on Buchman's work were invited to join four of the MRA Board of Directors, which up to then had been directing resources in support of *Up With People*. This opened the way for a fresh wave of relevant activity there.

In September, 1970, following extensive consultations with European colleagues, I was grateful to return to North America with Bill Jaeger, a man born into the working class of Northern England, who married an American, had travelled the world with Buchman and the work of Moral Re-Armament, and who knows labour and trade union leadership in every corner of the world. He had lived for years in North America.

People needed an explanation of what had gone wrong, what had happened to MRA as it had been known and understood. Many found that they had put their faith in a movement, and not foremost in God, and the thing that heartened them was to find that the work of MRA had in fact been steadily carrying on across the world, and that a lot of the things they had been told were not true. There had been no retrenchment.

Mitch Bingham, who owned the home where Buchman stayed in Florida, was one of the first Americans to work with Jaeger and myself in this task. His brother was a Member of Congress, his father had been a Senator, and his younger brother, Brewster, was also heart and soul with us. In Canada we worked very closely with Ted and Audrey Porter of Montréal, and with Drew Webster, of the noted Eastern Canadian Webster family, who had promised his father on his deathbed to continue his efforts to see that the money his father had earlier given to MRA was used for its intended purpose. This he did.

The net result was that Moral Re-Armament was re-launched in Canada and in the United States, in the early 1970s. It showed that there were a number of people who wanted to have a campaign of MRA, and the free use of the name Moral Re-Armament, and it restored the opportunity for all those who wanted to participate in the work of MRA as it had been known.

At the same time it was a critical stage in the life of the continent. In Québec the 'Front de libération québecois' (FLQ), had got to such a point of frustration that they had murdered a provincial cabinet minister, as part of their violent campaign against the English-speaking minority in Québec. In the United States people's heads and hearts were full of Vietnam, and then a few years later Watergate. There was a great bewilderment and sense of need in ordinary people, and to me there also seemed to be a clear strategy of evil which needed to be countered.

It seemed to bring into sharp focus the vigour and relentlessness of the will to destroy God's sovereignty. On most of my visits across the Atlantic Annejet remained in London, with our daughters.

(P to A)
September 18th, '70, NY

It seems more than a week since we left! We have not been idle. In NY people are on edge. In the lobby of our hotel early this morning a customer struck the news vendor in the face ... ... A militant Christian bid with the heart for people that God gives can win this nation to God's ideas.

September 27th, '70, NY

Bob Duffin, one of our good friends from Richmond, Va., has arrived with a Buick convertible which has added considerably to our mobility! Travelling in the subway here is like being placed in a baking oven with several hundred people hammering away on the outside!

October 5th, '70, NY

When I was in Detroit I had 45 minutes with my old friends the Sladens at the Henry Ford Hospital. He said it was a meeting of a life-time. It was an historic completion of a story that goes back 32 years!

He told me the hospital corridors are patrolled at night by men with dogs – it is not safe to step outside the hospital at night. The corridors of the General Motors head office are scanned by TV cameras – and the secretaries have to be escorted to their cars in the parking lot.

Do pray that we are steadily responsive to the Spirit's whispers. It does take a quiet mind and no preconceptions to hear the softly spoken word in your ear.

One evening in October, 1970, in Montréal, Dr Gustave Morf came to meet with Ted and Audrey Porter and others of us in the Porters' home. He was keen to talk over the situation in Québec, and to seek with us the wisdom of the Almighty on how best he could have an impact on it.

A Swiss doctor, he specialized in psychiatry, emigrated to Canada and became the psychiatrist for the prison service in Montréal and Québec. As such, he was the appointed psychiatrist for the FLQ men who were in prison. His book *Terror in Québec* is based on his interviews with them, and is internationally known for its clarity on the violence in Québec, and the reasons behind it.

(P to A)
October 14th, '70, Montréal

Half an hour after leaving us Dr Morf went on TV and radio nationally, on the FLQ and their kidnappings. He was excellent and brought reality and sanity. When asked how he explained it, he said, 'This type of action is the natural end-product of the permissive society.' He has been in touch with the leader of the opposition in Québec who was meeting with the Cabinet over the FLQ crisis. He wants to have René Levesque, the most prominent political separatist leader, see Bill Jaeger and myself. He feels MRA has something more revolutionary to offer these types.

October 29th, '70, Montréal

Morf plans to take me to the Federal Penitentiary tomorrow to visit an FLQ man who read *Refaire les hommes* (*Remaking Men*, the book I had written some years before). This FLQ man said, 'A wonderful book – bring me literature like that in any amounts.'

I believe one way to understand the Québec issue is to see it as Moscow's bid to control the St Lawrence valley and get a hand on the throttle of the heart of industrial America. They are trying to establish in that area an inland Cuba.

I was grateful for several far-ranging and helpful meetings with a man called Maurice Sauvé, whose wife later became Canada's first woman Governor-General. I first called on him in his office in Ottawa in 1964, when he was an MP from Québec. At that time I was introduced to him as being from MRA and he immediately tried to put me down. I asked him what he knew about Moral Re-Armament, and he said, 'Very little'. I replied that I was astonished that a man in his position could speak so freely on a subject he knew little about. We became firm friends.

He later held a Cabinet post under Trudeau, and on retiring from politics became an official of Consolidated Bathurst, a paper company. He sometimes came to breakfast with us in Montréal, where we found that he loves fresh croissants! After some conversation I would suggest a time of listening to the still small voice of Truth with which every human is equipped. And whenever we had interesting guests in town I took them to meet Maurice Sauvé.

The head of 2500 Port Workers in Montréal is called St-Onge. He refuses to speak anything but French in his Union office. The first time I met him was when an Irish friend, Eric Turpin, and I called on him at his office. We wanted to offer to show him the film *Les hommes du Brésil* (*Men of Brazil*). Everything we said was put into French by one of his men.

The film is a powerful and true-life story. One Rio dock-worker had brought his union rival, a man whom he had intended to murder, to see Buchman many years before. He said to Buchman, 'Till I met your people I had only two alternatives ahead of me – prison or a coffin.' The change in those two men made possible the first democratic and free union elections amongst Brazil's 10,000 dockers. It was their story, and that of their families, which was filmed, and it seemed to me to have relevance to our Canadian situation.

But St-Onge was not interested, not a flicker in his eyes. Then I said, 'My father came from Scotland, my mother from Yorkshire. In our home we had pictures of the Royal family and a big map on the wall with the British Empire marked out in red. I was brought up on Shakespeare and stories of Nelson and Wellington. I grew up with the idea that if you didn't have English blood in your veins you didn't quite measure up, and that those of us with English blood knew better and should be running things.

'Then I married a Dutch girl,' I continued. 'She has no English blood and what's more it doesn't bother her. One day she told me, "You don't think any ideas of mine are as good as yours." I didn't listen to her, but when she kept repeating it I realised it was my English superiority that was making me deaf. It explained my feelings towards the Americans, towards the French Canadians, and towards the Native people of our continent.'

Suddenly St-Onge came to life. He asked us to come and

show *Les hommes du Brésil* to his Executive Committee. And when we arrived at his Union Hall for the event, he greeted us in English at the door. It showed me that language is not the real problem, but it's a question of attitude.

When I phoned the head of the Port of Vancouver – who used to be in Montréal – to tell him about this event, he said, 'I am amazed you can even sit down with these men.'

A few days later St-Onge arranged for a further showing of the film for the Union men. Drew Webster spoke at the end of the film and really won them – saying his family had grown wealthy from the sweat of their fathers and grand-fathers. In those early days the ships brought in fire-bricks, a particularly rough substance to handle, even with gloves. As an incentive for the dockers to complete the job, the owners used to stack crates of whisky behind the bricks. Drew told his audience of dock-workers that he wanted his firm to aim not just at profit but to be part of the future of all the children of the Province.

Some years earlier I had been asked to address a meeting in Montréal, at which were gathered a number of young French-Canadian students just back from attending a conference at Mackinac, and the South American cast of the student play *El Condor*. At the end of the meeting, a young Montréaler came up to me, bristling with emotion. 'You're the sort of Englishman we can best do without,' he said to me.

Later he described the events as follows:

'You were introduced, and gave your talk. After the meeting some of us young Québecois gathered to share our reactions. We were all agreed that you had spoken with arrogance and superiority, without any understanding of the feelings in your audience.

'Personally I felt a certain amount of bitterness towards you. I could not put up with such behaviour, especially from an Englishman. To me you were the sort of "damned Englishman" we wanted to get rid of in Québec.

'After the meeting, with the help of an interpreter, I told you my feelings quite bluntly. I cannot recall exactly what you replied, but I do know that the more the conversation continued, the more I felt I had a different man in front of me than the one I had imagined you to be. Here was a man who listened, who apologized for his attitude of authority and arrogance, and for that of other English Canadians, and who had a challenge to give us.

'You brought to birth in me the conviction that every individual is important, and has a part to play in his country and in the world. I maintain to this day that prejudices fall away when people get to know each other. It is possible to build bridges, to have common projects, even if we come from different cultures.

'I was not a member of a nationalist Québec movement – just a young Québecois who was reacting to provocation by an Englishman. You must realise that for us at that time there were no English Canadians – only English.

'Thank you for the good times we have had together, and for the convictions you have planted deep within me.'

We became firm friends. He is working with the Provincial Police in Québec and we meet and talk every time we go to Montréal.

(P to A)
November 4th, '70, Montréal
    On Thursday evening Drew Webster was host to 20 of us at dinner with General Jean Victor Allard, former head of the Canadian Armed Forces, at the Engineers' Club in Montréal. This Club has a predominantly English-speaking membership, in the French-speaking city. As he came in the General – a French-Canadian – said to me, 'This is the first time I've been in this club!' It was an incident reminiscent to me of the way the British behaved in India for so long. He said, 'The reason I went for the leadership of the army was that I was determined to show that a French Canadian could do it!'

We had with us representatives of trade unions and management from British industry, men who had found a common purpose, commitment and understanding, when they might otherwise have been facing each other down across shop-floors and board-room tables.

General Allard was greatly impressed by Les Dennison – a plumber and trade union leader from Coventry, England, who had been captured by and suffered at the hands of the Japanese in Burma during the war. He had been a member of the Communist Party for 25 years until meeting the fundamentally different ideas of MRA.

Also with us was John Vickers, chairman of a lubricants manufacturing company in Yorkshire, England, who has a wealth of practical experience and evidence of a new spirit of co-operation at work in industrial management. These two men, speaking together, made quite an impact.

In addition to the many opportunities in Québec, I was grateful for numerous chances to visit Alberta and British Columbia, meeting old friends and making new ones.

(P to A)
November 1st, '70, Calgary

We have been meeting with several local Calgary friends, and they all felt they had, after a long time, been re-united with a world family and force. One woman said she had not slept after our evening's discussion – she was so thrilled with the developments.

The next day the Edmonton friends motored down and we had an excellent time together.

. . . Some Canadians suffer from the Canadian disease of feeling they don't count. Everything of importance happens somewhere else and by someone else. Not so our friends in the West.

In this country we need 1000 homes where people simply obey God's daily leading. You feel a new awareness in people of what it takes to get God in charge of a nation.

November 5th, '70 en route to LA from Vancouver

How you would have enjoyed this trip, and one day before long we will come with the children. Because of fog in Calgary we left at 1.00 pm on Sunday by bus for Victoria. What a marvellous journey through the Rockies – and a memory-tingling 15 minutes in Banff. Mitch Bingham and Bill Jaeger really loved it.

We were in Vancouver by 6.30 am Monday – having

gone near my town of Armstrong in the Okanagan en route to Kelowna (just nine miles away). We had a superb ferry trip and I could see Aunt Bertha's house on Salt Spring Island.

Before we left Calgary, one man gave me his old age pension cheque of $120 – several others pressed $10 and $20 into my hand. They thus covered the bus trip to Victoria, and our stay last night in Vancouver. I am continually grateful for and moved by such generosity.

March 25th, '71 en route to Montréal from Vancouver

Two veins of strategy – the construction industry and the maritime industry – seem to be God's way to have an impact on this country. We are being led to the men in Québec, Vancouver and the rest of Canada. We have been able to share our experiences and enlist them in building a network of people who would really care for Canada's future.

Yesterday morning we had almost two hours with Ed Strang, the President of the Waterfront Employers Association, whom I had earlier visited in his office in Vancouver, and his two chief aides. In the afternoon we had superb times with the top officials of the Building and Construction workers for BC and for Western Canada, to whom we were taken by local friends.

Mary Hamilton, a former teacher in Victoria, BC was 80 yesterday. Those senior ladies are in touch with the cabinet and the trade union leaders, for they were their pupils – it is quite unique in my experience. One woman said to Mary, 'Where, at your age, do you get your drive?' 'I have a purpose,' replied Mary.

I think you are right about not coming over at this point to join me – but if you don't come next time they won't let me in the country!

April 22nd, '71 Montréal

At the Victoria end of the ferry we were met by Superintendent (Royal Canadian Mounted Police) and Mrs McNeil, and taken to their home. Bill Jaeger and I met him for the first time when we all went out there early in

March. He has great fame for his work in the Arctic – with the dogsleds etc. He told us many hair-raising tales of life in the Arctic, and said that modern means of transport are fine, but if you were in danger of starving in the old days, you could at least eat the huskies! He was much interested in what we have been doing in Montréal, Trois-Rivières and Québec City since our last visit.

January 19th, '72 Montréal
Yesterday Drew and I had almost two hours, by appointment, with the head of security for RCMP in Québec, informing him about the work we have been doing.

To Roly Wilson and Lawson Wood, in London
In our affluent nations the greed-rate has exceeded the production-rate. We have come to the point where the freedom of everyone to demand what he wants cannot be tolerated much longer, without the collapse of society. . . . One of our aims here in Québec is to build up in the unions men who can effectively give a better leadership than is being given by either those who are for or those who are against the Establishment. A leadership which is out to change both.

Chapter Thirteen
OUR PROBLEM IS THIS BIG

IN THE LATE Sixties, I was invited to go and stay in Belfast by friends. It was the first of many visits, to both the North and South of the country. I met and made friends with a marvellously varied group of men and women, Protestant and Catholic, Orangemen and priests, as well as committed Sinn Fein. It was a rare privilege to be welcomed in so many homes.

For the first time I came face to face with the so-called 'Irish problem', and at the same moment was confronted with evidence of profound change which could be the 'Irish solution'.

There was Tommy, a Protestant metalworker, who told me, 'I didn't hate Catholics. I never met one.' But he did hate his boss with a passion. When he, with the help of friends, became free of this hatred, his eyes were opened to the fact that there was not a single Catholic employed in his factory. He began to see the injustice and he started to put it right.

Another friend, an architect, a Protestant, told me that in his firm when they advertised for personnel, they would look over the applications that came in and if there was a name or an address that indicated the person was a Catholic, it was automatically dropped in the waste-paper bin without even reading the person's qualifications. But recently, he said, he had decided to make a Catholic his business partner, because he felt this man was the best person for the job.

There were many other stories like that, so contagious, yet so simple. Regular evenings were held in a Belfast monastery for Protestants and Catholics to get to know each other, and become friends. Father McCarthy, a big-hearted priest from Limerick, won the confidence of these men and women.

Incidentally, it just so happens that many of my Irish friends and I share the same passion – golf! Annejet and I were invited for a magnificent holiday in Killarney, where the men played golf all day and Annejet could relax in the sun with a book. She is amazed how people like me can play so badly and yet enjoy it so much.

On another visit, this time to Dublin, I asked a Sinn Fein official, 'What is your aim?'

He answered, 'We want to unite the workers, the shop-keepers, the farmers in the North *and* in the South into a fist to smash the oppressors.'

I was interested to read that more than a century ago Karl Marx wrote that it would be impossible for class war to succeed in Britain as long as the classes united to look down upon the Irish.

In trying to tackle similar issues in Canada, a group of Canadians decided to invite men and women from Ireland to come and help us. They were able to raise their own fares – it was a question of faith and prayer in practice. In Canada, many people gave them hospitality and provided transport and meals.

The party of 14 from Northern Ireland and the Republic, including Catholics and Protestants from Belfast came to Canada at a time when the warfare in Ireland was used by many as proof that faith is irrelevant to solving the problems of division and hatred. But these people from Ireland embody evidence that the deepest hate and prejudice can be cured, small aims can be replaced with a concern for the people of the world, and that a passion to put right what is wrong in our society – each one beginning with himself – is the factor that can enable people to solve their problems without resorting to violence.

They brought with them a documentary play, based on the miracles of change of many of those in the party, and rooted in the reality of their situation at home. They presented it as a reading in towns and cities across Canada, and in Washington and New York.

In New York they gave their play-reading in the home of friends. Muriel Smith, the mezzo-soprano, was among those present. At the end of the reading there was a profound silence. Then she rose to her feet and said, 'You must make this into a film. We need the evidence you bring that people really can be different.'

I remember Tommy Elwood, one of the party, Deputy

Chairman of Shop Stewards in a Belfast metal factory, saying after a couple of days in Québec, 'When I left Ireland I thought our problem was this big,' – holding his hands wide apart. 'Now, after two days I see it is this big,' with his hands about six inches apart, 'because I see you guys also have problems.' He is an Orangemen, and often in those days wore Union Jack socks as proof of his allegiance.

Once, in the course of the Canadian travels, he was billeted of all places in the guest room of a Catholic convent. He was really worried, and quite genuinely feared he might be dead in the morning. He told me later that he had left a little trail of breadcrumbs to his room, so he would know the way out again if he had to make a quick dash for it in the middle of the night.

Another member of the same party was Jack Lavelle, a former Republican Labour Councillor, and chairman of Shop Stewards in Britain's largest union, the TGWU. As such, he came from the opposite end of the spectrum. To have two such men travelling together was electrifying.

The Vicar-General of Trois-Rivières, Mgr Denis Clément, said to them, 'I find in the text of your play that it is not enough only to change the systems, whether they be capitalist, socialist or others, but that the hearts of men must be changed and this is precisely the change that MRA brings.'

(P to A)
January 22nd, '72
. . . The urgent and pressing need here is for Québec to find and give the alternative to the class-war philosophy, and also to the tide of separatism which is rising. Somehow we seem to get drawn to the areas in greatest need. God's leading and timing have been superhuman. I realise his timing is rarely what mine would be – but it is integral to his plan – and his accuracy is amazing.

Early in January 1972, some of the dock-workers from South America who had made the film *Men of Brazil* were invited to help us in Canada. We asked them to come and tell of their experiences of turning the Rio docks from gang warfare into a profit-making business, with democratically-elected unions. We felt their stories had a particular relevance to our Canadian situation.

(P to A)
January 24th, '72
    The Brazilian dockers, together with Michel Sentis, a friend from Paris, had six hours of discussion with the President and officers of the Port Workers in Trois-Rivières, who now would like to see the Brazilians' film. This is a major advance. One of the Brazilians has begun to have much longer times of quiet in the morning before breakfast, and to think for Canada and America, and not just for the Port Workers in Rio.

The visits of groups from overseas, such as the Irish and the Brazilians, gave opportunities to meet many of the most influential people of the Province. We were able to inform them about the work we were doing.

(P to A)
January 28th, '72, Montréal
    Jean Vincent, the man in charge of the Philips company in Québec, had three hours at lunch yesterday with Bill Jaeger and myself at the Badminton Club. He moves in the same circles as the younger French leaders of the Province.

In February 1972 we arranged a dinner in Montréal for some of the leading personalities of the Province to meet and hear from Frits Philips, Annejet's father. It was an opportunity that many were eager to accept.

(P to A)
February 5th, '72, Montréal
    . . . The dinner at which your father will speak will be at the Ritz-Carlton here, for up to 30 men. St-Onge of the Portworkers says he will come, and Manet of the Stevedoring Company, and Chief Justice Gold. The editor of *Le Devoir* has indicated he will come if at all possible, René Levèsque has accepted, as have the former head of

the CBC and the head of the CBC of Québec. These men are the intellectual powers in the Province.

They have all been told that I am arranging the dinner and have been here with the work of moral re-armament. Jean Vincent of Philips was deeply moved by the new documentary film about Caux, and feels it would be just right as a finale to the dinner.

Do you have a good recipe for the pre-dinner cocktails, and at the dinner itself? We shall have a separate function for your mother that evening with some of the leading women of the area.

February 21st, '72, Montréal
Your recipes came today – many thanks.

It must be difficult for you with the power-cuts [during the miners' strikes of the infamous British 'winter of discontent']. We have a strike here by the snow-cleaners – consequently it is difficult to move about.

February 25th, '72 – Hotel Ritz-Carlton, Montréal
Darling – last night was quite superb. Your father did magnificently and gave unstintingly from 7.00 till after 10.30 pm, which was close to dawn for him. He had the wave-length of the men. Some were held up out of town by the snow, but the others all came. There was a great deal of discussion, followed by the Caux film, in French.

Your father spoke in French, and gave his conviction that labour and management need to work together to pioneer a new spirit in industry, and to meet the needs of the Third World. I sat next to the head man for 125 Employers Associations in Québec who said, 'The trade unions no longer want to negotiate before striking.' He sees two fine lines between society and the moment of truth. One is the enactment of special legal procedures like the present injunction which forces the snow cleaners to go back to work. The next is the enactment of special laws such as 'no strikes'. But then what do you do when the men refuse to obey the law? An illegal strike is more damaging than a legal one, for it means anarchy. So far, in our nations, society rejects anarchy – the only alternative these men see is dictatorship of one form or another.

He said, 'Brains can't do it, for human emotions run brains. And the only way you can deal with emotions is by force.'

Your father's straight-forward sharing of his experiences had a great impact on these men.

March 12th, '72, Montréal

Today is Mother's birthday. She would have been 100. I have enduring gratitude for her faith and merry spirit. I am only sorry she did not have the opportunity to know you and the children. But she does now.

A nurse who was with us on Saturday night in Trois-Rivières, on Tuesday with two of my friends opened her life and decided to be honest with her father, an alcoholic. He has had 24 jobs in 25 years.

March 24th, '72, Montréal

May all the fresh joy and sparkle of Easter be yours, and all the family in Eindhoven.

This past week Ted Porter and I had an excellent time with General Allard, a very good lunch with Yvon Dupuis, editor of *Le Défi* and an evening with the head of the Typographical union at the Porters'. Last night Laurent Gagnon and some of the young people from Trois-Rivières dropped in.

Without Ted and Audrey we would never have been able to do this kind of work in Montréal. Nothing is too much trouble for them, and often their house is bulging with visitors from overseas. Audrey is a wonderful hostess, and seems able to whip up a meal for a dozen people in no time at all.

It is hard to believe how blind and unaware the English-run companies are towards the French. They always choose their executives from the English rather than from the French; young (French) engineers are going into Hydro-Québec or Government service, rather than companies, because in an English-run company they know their promotion is limited – the advancements will invariably go to the English. No wonder there is such pressure for separation here. They are so boxed in by this attitude, blindness and practice. We have got to change the English business community – the trick will be to help the French to do it.

Jean Vincent told me that when he was in the Navy, many years ago, he was told by his superiors, 'Speak white'. Clearly they felt English was the right language for white men. We English Canadians have caused so many wounds we've not even been aware of.

On Saturday morning we go to Vancouver with Dr Gustave Morf. It will be primarily a chance for Morf to shed light on the situation in Québec for Western Canada, and we hope to meet many of the press, media and opinion-makers. After seeing as many Government and press people as we can with Morf in Vancouver, we get to Edmonton on Wednesday evening, where he will be on radio the next day.

March 26th, '72, Victoria

The Province is faced with a time as crucial as any in many years. Negotiations are in progress or are due for 1. the International Woodworkers, 2. the construction industry, 3. the Port workers, 4. the towboat operators. If any one of them had a strike, it would have a crippling effect.

We went straight from the airport at Vancouver to the home of the Chairman of the Port Employers, and had almost two hours with him, ending in a time of quiet reflection together. The man had two emergency calls while we sat with him in his home, on a Saturday morning.

Then we had lunch at the golf club – wonderful to see green grass, primroses, even a rhododendron, after so many weeks of snow only. We caught the 5 pm ferry for Victoria – a beautiful sail.

March 30th, '72, Edmonton

Gustave Morf is enjoying every minute. He realises by the interest of TV, radio and press, that he has something to give the country. A very good Sunday evening with 50 in the hotel in Victoria.

Morf had almost two hours on an open radio line, an interview with the *Victoria Times*, and an hour with the new Mayor who has a Ford sales business. He wants some of our films to be shown to his Council.

We had lunch with Bruce Hutchison, the former editor of the *Winnipeg Free Press*, whom I have known for many years, in his club, the Union Club. He has just been to Ottawa, Boston and Washington, but as we parted he said, 'This has been more informative and more interesting to me than anything I have heard in the last few months.' He feels the major issue facing us is that, at the present use of our resources of air, and water and material, and the increasing garbage and waste, in 100 years or less we could no longer be able to sustain life on earth. 'This underlines for me the truth of what you people have been saying for years.'

Bill Jaeger, Morf and I had one-and-a-half hours with the head of the 70,000 building workers. He started life in Liverpool. Breakfast yesterday brought together 42 men, eight from the Legislature, the Premier's representative, the Speaker, the Leader of the Opposition and five of his colleagues, business and labour men, educators, men from the Department of Indian Affairs – a magnificent time, Gustave ably fielded questions for almost an hour. It was an education and the challenge of a fresh perspective. We are in the radio studios as I write, where Gustave is doing masterfully. I have secured the attaché case with the combination dial lock, for which your father left me money in Montréal, for exactly the amount he had given me. I had no idea such a case is so convenient and so very satisfactory to work with. I am grateful.

Chapter Fourteen

DON'T SEND ME MONEY!

(Paul to Annejet)
December 3rd '72, Montréal

YESTERDAY Jean Vincent came for the afternoon. Jacqueline Pellerin motored from Trois-Rivières to be there and spoke to him from her heart. She shook him with her love for Québec and her vision. He could hardly speak. I have rarely seen a man so moved. You will recall that we met her first at the home of our good friends in Trois-Rivières, Charlie and Aileen Pelletier.

Jacqueline Pellerin is a remarkable French Canadian. She lives in Hertel, an inner-city area of Trois-Rivières which, in 1970, was run down, with unemployment of 39%, and crime a major problem. About 350 families – over 1200 souls – live in the area, surrounded by the port, a textile factory and a paper mill, the prison and the cathedral, a convent and City Hall.

In 1970 the city authorities produced a plan to raze the entire area, creating a site for a more lucrative development. It would have meant that families who had lived in the area for generations would have to move out and find other accommodation. The risk was that others might move in when the building was completed, and a community would be dispersed.

The local people were deeply opposed to the plan, and Jacqueline Pellerin, an ordinary mother of four, with very little formal education, became their leader. A social action committee (CASH – Comité d'Action Sociale Hertel), of which she was elected President, was set up to oppose the city's plans. They drew up proposals of their own with the help of various people, including a priest. She worked with organizations who provided clothing for the needy, and architectural students who created plans for new housing more suited to the existing community – some very large, for the big families, others small enough for a single senior citizen.

In the end it was agreed that the worst houses should be replaced by low-cost units, including a residence for senior citizens. Plans were drawn up for the many other properties which could be renovated. The city authorities found in Mme Pellerin a formidable adversary.

But then something changed in her approach. She went to Northern Ireland on a visit arranged by friends with Moral Re-Armament. It was, in a way, a return visit by Canadians to those who had come to Canada from Belfast and elsewhere in previous years. When she left Montréal, 55 of her friends from Trois-Rivières drove the 95 miles to see her off. The local radio station asked her to phone them, collect, from wherever she was, to tell them what she was doing. They offered to put her on air whenever she rang.

In Belfast she found situations even more painful than her own, but she also found an inner strength and a larger perspective from the people she met. The men and women of Northern Ireland, who had contributed so much in Canada, were generous in their hospitality and in sharing their faith and their experiences with their Canadian guests.

She travelled on to Caux, to attend the conference there, and then returned home saying, 'Of course we must renovate homes. But we must also renovate the people.'

On her return home, Jacqueline Pellerin began to work with lawyers and reporters, the Mayor and Member of Parliament, the police and welfare workers. She personally arranged new accommodation for those whose homes were to be rebuilt, reassuring those who would have to move out that the new house would actually be for them. Day care for the children was established, and some leisure facilities; unemployment and crime have begun to decline, and the community has learned to care for its own.

Her new attitude and spirit surprised the city authorities, and contributed to the credibility of the community's own proposals, when they were studied by the provincial and federal governments.

She said to the local MP, 'Don't send me money, I will

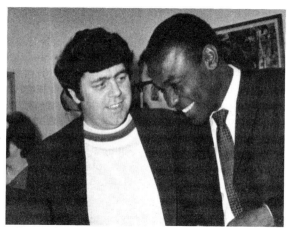

Tommy Elwood, of Belfast, and Conrad Hunte, the West Indian cricketer, in Trois-Rivières.

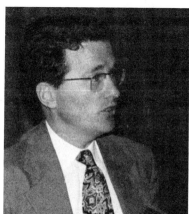

Drew Webster of Montréal.

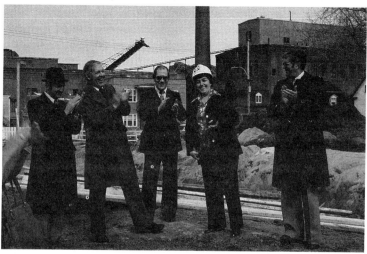

'Jacqueline Pellerin (second from right) is a remarkable French Canadian.' In the inner-city area of Trois-Rivières houses were rebuilt and renovated, tailor-made for each family.

send you our bills.' He replied, 'If everyone in Québec was as honest as you, we would save the Province a lot of money!'

When the citizens' plans were finally accepted by the authorities, funds were made available and housing units were tailor-made for individual families. They could even choose their neighbours.

(P to A)
December 9th, '72, NY
We had a superb time in Trois-Rivières with Mgr Clément, the Vicar-General – two hours. We had a time of quiet together. After which he said, 'We need a re-assessing of conscience before the situation of the Church. You know the pulse of the region. The whole of our life is involved. Where have we gone wrong?'

Then we had six hours, till 10.30 pm, with Jacqueline Pellerin and 60 of her people. They gave us supper.
We also had an evening in St Joseph's seminary. One Father was at Caux this last summer. The things that struck him during his three days there were: 1. the order and quality of the silence, 2. 400 people, no one smoking and no sign saying 'no smoking', 3. the availability of people to help you, with no sense of trying to possess you, 4. the small book for making notes during one's time of listening to the inner voice – the ease with which people can speak of self without pride.

One thing life with Buchman taught me was never to lose sight of the fact that our main work is with individual people. You cannot hope to straighten out the life of a Province or of a nation if you don't deal with the needs of individual people. Only God can lead you to the heart of another person's life. But you have to be ready for it.

(P to A)
October 9th
Last night a husband and wife had me to dinner and the evening to talk over their life together. They gave me artichokes and steak!

She demands and shouts and he reacts in like manner.

150

She said she noticed their child got very quiet when they were shouting. I said, 'Of course – the child is terror-stricken at such times.' I would say that that illumination went deeply into her tough hide – both heart and conscience. I was there till midnight.

They seemed to get the point that the centre of their life is meant to be not the child or their own relationship but the needs of America.

We were quiet together, and his thought was, 'When we are right with God we will be put on parallel tracks. I have new hope. Renew morning prayer and time of listening to God. The only demands you make must be on yourself. Learn to disagree without being disagreeable.'

March 20th

There was a real slanging and shouting match Saturday evening in our friends' home till 12.30 am. The idea that caught their imagination was that the only way to end a cat and dog fight was for both to chase the same rabbit!

His insensitivity, making her feel 'like a trapped animal', his smoking when he knew he should stop, his drinking, and what she feels are bad manners – and her constant nagging on these points – had him saying he couldn't put up with it any longer, and divorce was the only way.

Much that was wrong with her went back to an affair she had not been honest with him about. This I encouraged her to do. She was really petrified, because if divorce came her admission would mean he would get custody of the child. But she did tell him. He was quite marvellous and 'big' in his response. From then on she looked 15 years younger and all tension went out. It was merry.

Last night, after a very good dinner, he said they had been getting their troubles out of all proportion, in relation to the needs of the country and of their friends. 'The how and why of helping the country will become clear. I can see the vision unfolding. We have to do it. If we don't we can't expect anyone else to.'

The thought of living without demand is, for her, a

terrific challenge, and could be her road to faith and a new life.

I followed all the childrens' activities at home and at school as closely as I could. Edith Anne and I have a good rapport, in that we both like to study. I used to rejoice in exams, because it gave you a chance to review everything you were supposed to know.

And Edith Anne and I love reading the same books – P G Wodehouse, for example, laughing out loud, and Shakespeare and others.

(P to A)

March 15th, '72, Montréal

Thank you for sending EA's report. She certainly takes after her grandparents. It is really satisfactory – her steady improvement and reliability. Do you know if her question on how to describe my occupation is cleared up for her? She will know how best to do it, if she thinks about it with us. Her definitions must satisfy her and be intelligible to her friends. The fact is that I am a doctor who works in many parts of the world. I practice the medicine of the future – an advanced type – but that is another matter.

I was pleased to have the picture of Digna's three kings, three camels and the crib. Carry on drawing! The kings and camels look very happy.

February 14th, '73

Hi Valentine,

Is Digna on the pink anti-histamine medicine? It might help her over this period. I hope she doesn't have enough will-power to develop a cold just to stay home! ... ...
I hope EA will write me how *Treasure Island* finally ends. It is a fascinating story.

There is no food on this plane. We left at 12.45 and get in at 1.45 – the airlines are economizing – on my stomach!

I am reading a book on the poor way the Dutch handled their North American colony. The rascals were more intent on getting profit than in developing the colony, so they lost both. Wall Street got its name from the road that ran along the wall on one side of the colony.

The times when we were able to have the children with us in Canada, during their Easter or Christmas holidays, for example, gave them a natural feeling of what I did when I wasn't home, and the people who were our friends. There were such contrasts in the homes we were invited to stay in – the wonderful home of ex-Ambassador Fred Bull, who had been posted both in Holland and Japan as Canada's Ambassador, with the special delight of its indoor pool; and then the family from India we stayed with in Trois-Rivières, the four of us in one room, climbing over our suitcases to get to the door. Sometimes we stayed at the convent in Trois-Rivières, where we got to know the nuns, and of course often in Montréal with Ted and Audrey Porter – such a warm-hearted couple with four children of their own.

Other friends lent us their country place just outside Ottawa for a family holiday. In the house there was a chest of dressing-up clothes, and the girls had a wonderful time acting out scenes from *The Little House on the Prairie*. It was a wonderful old farmhouse, with quilted blankets, and when the pipes all froze we had to get snow from outside and melt it on the stove. Indeed it felt like the pioneering days.

(P to A)
April 25th, '73, Vancouver
I was sorry to see the three of you on your way after such wonderful days. I hope you had a good trip.

April 30th, '73, NY
Saw Nixon on TV this evening on the Watergate case. How accurate Buchman was, that unless men change men they cannot rule well. It seems here that the only evil is to be caught.

The Watergate case seems to find its significance in the fact that it is not an isolated incident, but an exposure of a practice that is widespread. It is just the way things are being done.

November 26th, '73 en route Montréal by train

I called Frank Sladen Jr and his mother on Thanksgiving Day. My old chief had died the previous Saturday. All the family were together and having a memorial service the next day. It was a most timely call. I also wrote Catherine (Mrs Sladen) a letter of appreciation for what they had both meant to me. The building together of a world force is as important as anything else we do. God's weapon for the world.

. . . It seems to me following Peter Howard's death and the point at which many of the Americans, Germans, Japanese, Brazilians, and Danes took a different road, we began to look inward as a force – quite understandable, but none the less wrong. The Westminster Theatre and Caux gave us a way of keeping the momentum going, while still being concerned with the world, and above all busy.

. . . A basic thing that has been wrong in recent years in our work is that too many of us were committed to an activity, a programme, an idea, but not basically to God and his will for the world, regardless of failure or calumny or hardship. Answering human need as, for instance, in Ireland and Québec is the greatest force for unity and change given to man.

December 3rd, '73 en route Edmonton to Montréal

Bruce Hutchison, just back from Washington and Boston, said 'Your diagnosis and understanding of affairs has been abundantly proven by recent events. The people in Washington are so engrossed in solving immediate problems (Watergate) that no one takes time to think.'

We have had marvellous times in Vancouver, Victoria and Edmonton.

Chapter Fifteen

THE SHAMROCK
AND THE PEACE-PIPE

AFTER BEING AT home with the family in London over Christmas in 1973, I returned to Canada early in 1974. The partings did not get any easier, but Annejet and I were both at peace, knowing it was part of the work to which we felt called.

I have not been paid a salary since I left the Henry Ford Hospital. Buchman never gave me any money, though he did share his meals with me when we stayed in a hotel. But there has always seemed to be enough money to go around. A lifetime has taught me that where God guides you to go, he also provides the means to make it possible.

Many Canadians send us gifts, often from their pensions – and when we go to Canada we very often stay as the guests of different families.

(P to A)
March 9th '74, Montréal
   Skies are blue and sun shining brightly and practically all the snow gone – although there can be big storms this month.

March 18th, '74
   Last Sunday evening 17 of the Calgary people met for a get-together, including Chief David Crowchild, his wife Daisy and son Gordon Crowchild. We had a truly excellent evening.
   Chief David apologised to another man for having excluded him. He said he'd believed this man was against him because of the work he does with the Indian Affairs (government) Department.
   Another man talked to me about what I had said of

the quiet-time as being in part a time of feeding on the Bible, and not just making something of a laundry list of things to be done. He said he would start listening to God again on that basis. Six feet of snow in Edmonton – not so much in Calgary.

There is certainly a warm welcome for us as a family in these parts. I think we shall have to come at least as far as Alberta, or we won't be forgiven.

April 10th, '74, Montréal

A general strike hits us here tomorrow, and there is no saying how long it will last.

The forthcoming conference in Alberta comes 40 years after Frank was made a blood brother by Chief Walking Buffalo. Chief Bill McLean, his son, may give us an evening meal on the Reserve next Sunday.

May 22nd, '74, NY

Americans are deeply frustrated, angry, pained and bewildered by Vietnam. I feel for those mothers and fathers and wives who have lost sons, husbands, fathers, and they might well ask, 'To what purpose?' Whatever the outcome, the problems of Asia remain. That is the key, the changing of people in key positions. Our task, I am convinced, is not to save a crumbling civilisation, but to build a new one. We are like David and Goliath – but David won. He hit Goliath in the mind and bigness collapsed.

May 24th, '74, Montréal.

My schedule is as follows. Tomorrow Montréal to Victoria, for dinner Monday evening; Tuesday Victoria to Edmonton, for a breakfast in Edmonton Wednesday morning; Friday to Sunday night June 2nd, in Calgary at the conference; June 3rd Calgary to Montréal, and Montréal to London, arriving 10.15 am June 5th!

May 30th, '74, Calgary

How are you all? I cannot wait to get back. I seem to miss you all so much.

The Gowards were generous in their hospitality, including a pastel of my wife's husband, which Elizabeth will send. It will need to be behind glass or it will smudge. (The subject matter may necessitate it being behind the cupboard door!) Had a good time in Victoria.

The Mayor of Victoria was a surprise, but typical. Quite sure people need a faith for social cohesion, but said, 'Do you think the mra we need is Chinese Communism?' This is the Achilles heel in our Christian west – the gap between personal faith and the way to build a new society. It is the nominal Christians' woolly thinking. My! What a fundamental contribution Buchman made to the human family.

Last night some of us had an hour with Chief Bill McLean and his wife Caroline at the Morley Reserve. He says he has just begun to see what his father, Walking Buffalo, did for his people.

October 17th, '74, Montréal

The trees are deep reds and golds and browns, and gaily clapping their hands – as Isaiah has it. The skies are blue and sunny.

In 1974 over 100 people contributed to the purchase of a house in the French-speaking part of Montréal, to be used as a centre for the re-established work of Moral Re-Armament in Canada. Annejet and I were both present at the luncheon marking the opening of the centre, as were Annejet's parents, Frits and Sylvia Philips, and many long-standing friends from all over Canada, as well as dignitaries from the city and the Province.

Speaking at the luncheon, Frits Philips said, 'Today everything is failing. It may well be the time when people will open their hearts to find what to do. This does not mean an instant universal solution, for the answer works in individuals. But when we accept it, we get right attitudes and make right decisions. When people do that they have a wide influence – wider than they know.'

We had another group from Northern Ireland and the Republic come on a three-week visit to North America, this time bringing with them the newly completed documentary film made about their experiences, *Belfast Report*. They visited 15 cities on the continent, and had 37 showings of the film.

(P to A)
October 28th, '74, Richmond, Va,

This morning our folk from Ireland are with the Mayor. We have a TV programme in Baltimore on Thursday, a meeting at the National Press Club on Wednesday, and see the head of the negotiators for the coal-mining operators on Thursday. A showing of the film on Capitol Hill for administrative aides on Wednesday, and a session at the State Department on Friday.

The pace is beyond that at which our friends normally move in Ireland. As always it focusses commitment – a very good thing.

Father McCarthy, one of the Irish party, has touches with the charismatic movement but says they have no strategy. In what we do he finds 'the structure for applying Christianity practically to our affairs' as nowhere else.

... Our hosts in Philadelphia were the supporters of the IRA. The film rocked them, as did the joint presence of the Orangemen and Father McCarthy. Whereas at the beginning they felt the only valid programme of action was to work for a united Ireland, and the British army was the enemy, the message got through that without the changes in attitude which the visitors were living, there would be no solution of any kind.

... One Congressmen said to the Irishmen who visited him, 'You have worked out a moral and spiritual answer. On that we should be able to bring a political solution.'

... In Vancouver, we will see the head of the grain handlers, have a TV interview, a public session at the University, press interview, and a chance to see the wheat pool operators. Tuesday in Edmonton there are several functions, including a Parliamentary breakfast.

November 5th, '74

Our Irish friends are adjusting to the pace, and beginning to joke about it, which is a good sign!

Once, in Montréal, a group of them were in an elevator, leaving someone's office after an interview. Faced with a panel of control buttons the man closest to them said, 'What shall I press for the ground floor?'

Someone at the back of the elevator said, 'Press "RC".' (rez de chaussée/street level)

The fellow by the buttons, a Protestant Orangeman, retorted, 'I'm pressing no "RC" button for no man,' and they all ended up in the basement.

(P to A)
November 7th, '74

We showed the Irish film in the Indian Association offices in Edmonton, and had an excellent time there with Don and Harold Cardinal and Fred Gladstone. Some of the group had lunch with the Edmonton Labour Council Executive, and we had an excellent breakfast with 20 of the MPs, including the Minister of Transport. On Sunday evening there is a showing of the film at the university, with a good crowd including TV people.

Last night we saw the Northern Lights on our way home from the rodeo, where there had been ten-year-old boys bareback riding wild cattle!

November 11th, '74

Father McCarthy was a real win in Trois-Rivières – a great stroke for that city. Another of the Irish, Jim McIlwaine – deputy convenor at a Belfast engineering works and from the extreme Protestant right wing – said for the first time how in his heart he had despised the Catholics, and apologised publicly to McCarthy. It was the highlight of the evening.

The Irish gave encouragement and perspective to people in each city they visited. This may even have been one of their greatest services to the North American continent.

(P to A)
May 5th, '75 NY

On Friday evening we will be in Baltimore for the

159

weekend with upwards of 30 of our most convinced people on this side of the country. The aim is to seek together how to get MRA as such in full flood, when the national need for it has never been more obvious. Watergate and Vietnam are powerful factors in people's search for an answer. And MRA is the essence of the principles and faith of the Founding Fathers.

May 16th '75, Richmond

We visited some of those whom the Irish had met, including a coal operator who had originally opposed the Irish visit to Rotary, because he was antagonistic to our friend Richard Brown. (Richard Brown is the black Academic Dean of Bluefield College, Virginia.) This coal operator said to Richard on Wednesday, 'I have been a racist – I apologise' and the two shook hands over his desk as we sat there.

Some time earlier Richard found himself with four white staff who were determined to get rid of him. He would come home cursing, 'I hate those men, I'd like to shoot them.' Then in a time of quiet meditation he had the simple thought – 'You can't control how you feel. You can determine how you deal. Treat those four men so that an observer would say "they must be among his best friends".' Inside four months they were. And he enjoyed doing it. They were so amazed at his change in attitude that they were drawn to him. It has transformed the spirit of the college and affected the community. I think I must take a leaf out of Richard Brown's book. It must apply to my attitude to everyone. . . . When we feel frustrated it is inside us. They are our feelings, and it is our choice how we react to the people and events around us. We can watch our feelings objectively and maintain our serenity at the heart of our being. We must not let events around us dictate how we feel.

It gives me great freedom of heart, for which I am grateful.

Annejet joined me in Banff, Alberta in June, 1975 – for the first major MRA assembly in North America for many years.

160

At Banff, where the Bow River carries water from the Rockies on to the vast expanse of the prairies, over 340 people from all over the North American continent, and with delegates from 16 other countries, gathered on the theme, 'Canada and the United States, partners in a world task'.

Prime Minister Trudeau cabled a message, as did Alberta's Premier. From overseas there were black and white from South Africa, Maori and white from New Zealand, a senior diplomat from South East Asia, and many others including Irish men and women.

Four chiefs of the Sarcee and Stoney tribes welcomed the delegates. Chief David Crowchild opened the conference. He recalled the occasion in 1934 when Frank Buchman was made a blood brother of the Stoneys by Chief Walking Buffalo.

Chief Bill McLean said, 'I am taking the responsibility of my late father, Walking Buffalo . . . I used to be very superior to other people, and had very bitter feelings toward the white people. Now we need to stand together and fight for what is right.'

Chief John Snow of the Stoneys added, 'The Great Spirit put us on this continent for a purpose. We must once again listen to the voice of the Great Spirit.'

Chief Gordon Crowchild of the Sarcee said, 'The first time I went to a conference like this was in 1958 at Mackinac when I was a wild young whipper-snapper. I had a lot of ideas, but I didn't have the right idea. I know that it is a challenging world, but if a person has the knowledge and guidance of God in whatever he does in his decisions, it makes a lot of sense in your leadership or whatever position you hold.' There was a delegation of 26 from Québec, both French and English speaking.

John Bocock, a member of the new MRA Board in Canada, and co-manager with his brother of a 1500-acre dairy farm near Edmonton, told of action he had taken to build trust between the farmers and the Vancouver grain-handlers. This was at a time when Canadian farmers were reportedly losing millions of dollars because of strikes by the grain-handlers.

At the final session, Chief John Snow came to the platform in full regalia. He said he wanted to re-establish the link that

161

was made with Frank Buchman in 1934. He presented me with a Pipe of Peace, and gave me the name 'White Cloud'.

It is an honour conferred on few white men, and one which touched me deeply. In responding to the Chief I said I believed that North Americans needed to become 'a people who listen to the Great Spirit in the home, in the executive meeting, in the trade union council and in the city council, in the Provincial and Federal government. On that basis we will have the birth of a new type of civilization.'

(P to A)
Summer '75, Caux
2 marvellous tennis games with your father – yesterday's with Bunny (Austin) and Bremer (Hofmeyr). Your Dad thoroughly enjoyed them. We have a return match on Thursday.

A senior Swiss colleague, Henrik Schaefer, tells me this evening that there are several Paul Campbells – some he knows better than others . . . the father and husband, the doctor, the actor, the man who feels he must move things forward – and he would like to see them more thoroughly integrated! . . .

I talked with Fred here, who has been getting clarity about his children. He has tried to maintain order at home by using his temper and has reaped a reign of terror. He is going to ask the childrens' help.

August 26th, '75, Caux
Chief David Crowchild's son Arnold, together with his wife Regena, have arrived here – he says I am a Chief! He said I must not underestimate the significance of the gift of the Peace Pipe Chief John Snow gave me at Banff – which is a most prized possession.

Some weeks later I found myself back in Canada once again.

(P to A)
October 4th, '75, Calgary
We had Thanksgiving dinner (turkey, pumpkin pie), then Jack flew in from Edmonton, and then the Crowchilds – Arnold and Regena, Gordon and Marie, and

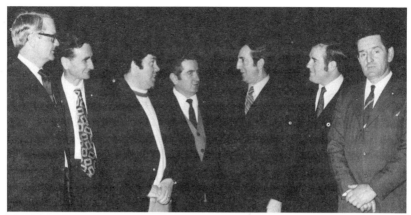

The Irish delegation with the Mayor of Trois-Rivières.

Chief John Snow presented me with a Peace Pipe at the Banff conference in 1975, and gave me the name 'White Cloud'.

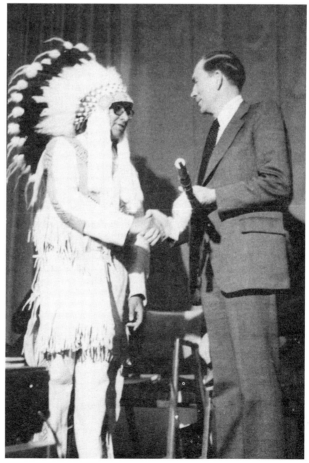

Leonard Crane – came in to meet with others. We men sat on the floor. A truly marvellous evening.

It seems to me our work is simply to obey the Spirit. So often I aim at results, but then it may be my aim and not God's.

October 5th, '75, Concord, Massachusetts
18th wedding anniversary

Lovely weather here, and the trees beautiful in colour. Concord is where the British had a rough time with the local farmers who potted them from behind trees.

I am grateful for God's great gift and goodness over these 18 years. The richest of my life.

October '75 Montréal

Magnificent hours here with a man of about my age who had been a close colleague and friend during Buchman's lifetime, but had chosen to walk a separate path in recent years. He said he had looked to Buchman for ideas and direction, then to Peter Howard, then to the next generation amongst his own countrymen, and no longer knew what he himself thought. I think it is true. Some people were driven by every strong wind, and when someone whom they regarded as being 'in charge' said 'say this', they said it, or 'go', they went. My friend says what is needed is the steel of an irrevocable commitment to the Almighty, regardless of anyone else.

October 6th, '75 Boston

Yesterday morning we went to the First Baptist Church. It was Communion Sunday which, with certain hymns, always moves me deeply. For me, faith in Christ is the deepest experience of the human heart – and I think through the Service faith is revealed to me for what it really is – the reality of Christ and his love for me, and of course it is associated with the simple devotion of my father and mother. Anyway something goes on inside me which I don't fully understand, but for which I am grateful. Anything that can melt the old human heart in this day is valuable.

October 18th, '75, Edmonton

Today Digna celebrates her birthday – it is already 3 pm with you, so the outing should be in full swing.

My goodness, God is good. Of course, he has his plan for the nation, and all we have to do is do what he says and the plan unfolds. We don't have to cook up a new world ourselves.

Chapter Sixteen

THE CHIEFS OF TREATY #7

ARNOLD AND REGENA Crowchild sat down together one day during their visit to Caux in the summer of 1975, to talk about their lives, and to be honest with themselves about the state of their marriage. Regena later said, 'We decided that it was a time for us to change. We had fooled people, bringing out the good side of ourselves. Life was not all rosy after that, but it was different. We learned that we were put in this world to care for each other, not to judge one another.'

Arnold put it another way, 'Because of my selfishness, and my arrogance and everything else, we would have split up eventually. We would have said, "To heck with it. We'll throw in all the chips and forget it." But in my wife and my three girls I have a lot to be grateful for. And I said to myself, "OK, I'm going to do something for my country".'

In January 1976 Arnold organised a conference in Calgary, entitled 'Native Conscience Re-Strengthening'. Present were Chiefs and senior representatives of the five tribes of Treaty #7 – signed in 1877 between Queen Victoria and the native peoples of Southern Alberta.

In calling for the conference, Arnold said, 'The time has come to move away from the wrongs of the past, to unite all races, to be responsible for our land and every creature upon it. Anything smaller than this will be too small to be worth fighting for, and division will multiply as we think only of ourselves.'

At the opening meeting, following an invocational prayer in his native language by Chief David Crowchild, the Mayor welcomed delegates to his city. Ed Burnstick, Canadian director of the militant American Indian Movement (AIM), was one of those present, and his speech was reported in the *Calgary Herald* next day. He said, 'Violence between Canada's Native people and white society will only continue to grow unless there is a change in attitude by both sides. . . . (MRA) is the only group of people I have ever come across who can really understand the world problems and understand people, and are determined to work and try and solve some of these problems.'

An AIM colleague, Nelson Small Legs Jr, added, 'I speak to many audiences, and the spirit of criticism in them is such that I am always speaking on the defensive. Here there is a kind of spirit of goodwill such as I have never experienced. It changed my whole attitude.'

Mrs Grace Young of Ottawa said, 'The thing that hit me about this conference invitation, and challenged me to come, was that this is a conference for Indians and non-Indians. I had never thought of myself as a non-Indian. Perhaps for the first time in our lives as white people we have taken the chance to sit down and really listen and understand what is going on in the hearts of the Native Canadians.'

I was asked to speak. I said, 'I want to bring the most profound change, not only to Calgary, to Alberta, to Canada, but to the entire world. I am against violence. I think it is morally wrong. It slows down the process of change. Violence hardens the hearts of the people against whom it is committed. I crave this passion for change – but change based on absolute honesty, purity, unselfishness and love. Change needs certain moral and spiritual content and direction in this age.

'I see a tremendous destiny for the Native people of Canada, who could share a way of bringing change swiftly, a change in which everybody benefits and no one loses. I want to see men fighting for that change with clean hands and pure hearts, and a concern not just for their own people, but for the whole of suffering humanity. Not a new organisation or denomination, but a new determination.'

At the final session each Chief of Treaty #7 spoke.

Chief Bill McLean of the Stoneys, son of the late Chief Walking Buffalo, said, 'I think we have come to a turning point. . . . believe God has put us here on this continent with a purpose. We need to stop once in a while to listen to the Great Spirit and live what he tells us. If we Indians live this, we can change the white man, the people, our government and North America.'

Fred Gladstone, President of Kainai Industries on the Blood Reserve, whose father had been the first of his people to sit in the Canadian Senate, said, 'With the natural philosophy of the Indian people and their religion, MRA is a programme that I have to take a real good look at.'

Then Chief Gordon Crowchild of the Sarcee, Arnold's brother, rose on behalf of his fellow Chiefs of Treaty #7 to invite the MRA musical presentation *Song of Asia* to Canada.

Song of Asia, a marvellous spectacle of music, colour and movement, was created at the MRA centre, Panchgani, in India, by young men and women from all over Asia and the Pacific. In sketches, songs, true stories, and in dance it portrayed a tapestry of Asia's glory and tragedy, humour and heartbreak, and above all the belief and evidence of an answer to suffering, hunger, poverty, corruption and hatred.

It was a powerful and moving drama, performed by about 30 people from a dozen Asian and Pacific nations, who had travelled widely through India and South East Asia, and more recently across Europe. Arnold and Regena Crowchild had seen the presentation at Caux a few weeks earlier, and got to know the cast, and become fired with the vision of what this group could do for their people and for Canada.

The invitation was signed by Chief Gordon Crowchild, Chief Bill McLean, Chief of the Bearspaw Band of the Stoneys, Chief John Snow of the Wesley Band of the Stoneys, Councillor Nelson Small Legs of the Piegan Tribe, Chief Leo Pretty Young Man of the Blackfoot, and Fred Gladstone of the Blood Tribe.

The invitation read:

'Together we can restore respect to people and a love of nature so that the hungry are fed, the oppressed are set free and we are led not to greed for gain but by the wisdom of the Great Spirit, the God of all people.'

The Native people of North America have a saying, 'Do not criticize a man before you have walked a mile in his moccasins'. In the weeks based in Calgary, the *Song of Asia* group who arrived in May 1976 were privileged to share experiences with the Native people which few others in the world today will have had. It began with the reception at Calgary Airport. All the Chiefs of Treaty #7, in full regalia,

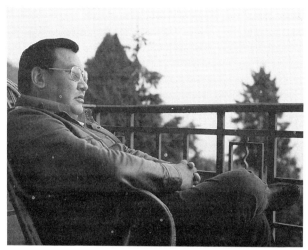

Arnold Crowchild at Caux 1975 decided, 'I'm going to do something for my country.'

The Chiefs of Treaty #7 at Calgary Airport: (l to r) Chief John Snow, Stoney Reserve; Acting Chief John Chief Moon, Blood Reserve; Chief Gordon Crowchild, Sarcee Reserve; Councillor Nelson Small Legs Snr, Piegan Reserve; Chief Leo Pretty Young Man, Blackfoot Reserve; the Hon Ralph Steinhauer, Lt Gov of Alberta; Chief David and Mrs Crowchild, Sarcee Reserve.

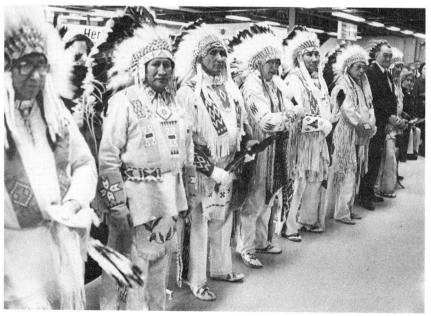

and Lt Governor Ralph Steinhauer, himself a Cree Indian and Canada's first Native Lt Governor, received them in the arrivals hall. No one, except the British Royal Family, has ever had such a welcome to Canada.

Arnold Crowchild called a briefing session, soon after their arrival, to tell the group his hopes for the months ahead, and share with them and the rest of us what he felt for his people, their past and their future.

'Culturally an Indian is defined by his attitude to the Creator, his creation and his creatures,' he said to them. 'The things that are really important in the days ahead are that attitudes must change, between Indian and non-Indian. Your job is to bridge that gap. When the Chiefs of Treaty #7 give *Song of Asia* they give hope to this land. Do not be afraid of the truth. God is real – use him.'

A man from the Indian Affairs Department later told Arnold that in his view MRA provided the only common ground between the government, the Chiefs and the militant men in the American Indian Movement.

The group met many of the leading citizens of Calgary – in one day they met the Mayor, the chief of the city Police and spent time at the head office of the Alberta Wheat Pool. This was followed by a gala evening at the Convention Centre in down-town Calgary, to which came all the Treaty #7 Chiefs and their wives, and the Lt Governor of Alberta, the Hon Ralph Steinhauer, and his wife, and 700 others. Many Calgarians commented that they had never seen the Chiefs treated with such respect and dignity at any function in the city. Each one was welcomed onto the stage by the cast, and given a gift and some flowers. Chief John Snow of the Stoneys said at the end of the performance, 'It is appropriate to restate a saying by Chief Walking Buffalo who toured the world with MRA, and perhaps visited many of your countries. He used the analogy of a beautiful forest, made of various trees, plants, ferns, colours. There are straight trees and tall trees, crooked trees and short trees, trees of all colours – trees that are red, black, white and yellow. And so all together they make a beautiful forest, and one of the secrets is because they live in harmony with one another; they live in accordance with the plan of the Great Spirit. I am sure that we, as various peoples, cultures and languages can also make a beautiful forest of people all over the world.'

Following that evening the group went to almost all the Treaty #7 reserves around Calgary, and were royally treated everywhere they went. More and more we who travelled with them came to realise the truth of the old saying, that it is character that counts, and what use you make of your background and experiences, for the sake of others.

Included in the *Song of Asia* group were refugees from Laos and Vietnam, some of whom had lost family members in the war; young Maoris from New Zealand eager to exchange experiences with the Native Americans; men and women from Papua New Guinea, India, Taiwan, Philippines, Malaysia, Japan, Hong Kong, Turkey, Australia, and a representative of the Sami (Lappish) people of the Nordic North. Each one had much to offer their hosts, in terms of their own experiences, background and personality, and through the songs and scenes of their show, but they also found themselves learning a very great deal from the wisdom and traditions of their hosts.

A welcome addition was a group from Ireland, hosts in previous years to Canadians and Americans, including Chief Gordon Crowchild – part of the continuing interchange across the Atlantic. A Protestant couple from Belfast came with a Catholic friend. Billy Arnold, the Protestant, was master of an Orange lodge, and Mrs Annie McGowan is a Catholic and staunch Republican. Mrs McGowan told the group how Mrs Arnold had helped her to become reconciled with her own daughter. Dr Roddy Evans, a Protestant from the Republic of Ireland, speaking of the situation back home said, 'The mixture of a guilty conscience and self-righteousness are a most dangerous combination. It takes grace to allow others to come and help you. North America has done this for the Irish.'

The Sarcee Reserve lies on the south-west border of the city of Calgary. One of the main roads of Calgary is named Crowchild Trail, after Chief David Crowchild. But within a few feet, at the edge of the city, the hard-top road gives way to a different world – the home of the Sarcee people. At first sight the land is poor – dusty beyond belief, with only a few scrubby trees to give protection from the wind that blows off the Rocky mountains. Yet within a week of the first visit there of the *Song of Asia* group, spring had come and things were steadily turning green all round. And in every season the Rockies are a majestic backdrop to the land.

The Crowchild family, known and respected throughout Alberta, were true hosts to the 35 young Asian and Pacific men and women, escorting them on every occasion, teaching, guiding, and making us roar with laughter. One story Arnold Crowchild told was about the two white hunters lost out in the hills. They came upon a Native man sitting under a tree at the roadside, and asked him the way. The man replied that he didn't know. The white men asked how they could find someone to direct them. The Native man replied that he didn't know. The white men said, 'Oh, what a stupid fellow we've got here.'

The response was swiftly given, 'Well, I may be stupid, but I'm not lost!'

Arnold and Regena had the four young Maoris from *Song of Asia* staying in their home for over two weeks – not as guests so much as part of the family. Edwin Crane, Arnold's half-brother, policeman on the Sarcee Reserve, took time off to be at the rehearsals and meetings, the appointments in the city and visits to the other Reserves. His friendship, ever-ready humour, frankness and depth of understanding were greatly appreciated.

The first weekend after the group arrived in Canada we were all invited for a barbecue and some fresh air to Arnold and Regena's home. It had been intended as a relaxing afternoon, with a chance to talk and get to know each other. News came suddenly of a serious bush fire on one corner of the Reserve, and all able-bodied men took off in every available means of transport to fight the fire. It meant a great deal to the Sarcee people to have the Asian men working shoulder-to-shoulder with them at this time of very real need. One man from North-East India was affectionately dubbed a 'Black-foot Indian' . . . he had fought the fire barefoot.

Chapter Seventeen

BREAKING THE CHAIN OF HATE

ON A SUNNY spring morning the whole *Song of Asia* group took the Trans-Canada Highway west out of Calgary and drove towards the snow-capped Rockies. I was invited to accompany them. Soon there was nothing to be seen of the concrete and steel of the down-town city behind, and only the mountains in front, as far as the eye could see.

A few hundred yards off the highway, and we were on the land of the Stoney people, allocated to them a century ago by Queen Victoria's government at the rate of a square mile per family. It lies right at the feet of the Rockies, the land of Tatanga Mani – Chief Walking Buffalo – who became a legend among his people in his own lifetime. In the quietness you feel the closeness of nature and its Creator.

Chief John Snow, Chief of the Wesley Band, is a tall, bespectacled, slow-spoken man, with the traditional braids of his people, and a buckskin jacket embroidered with beads. He welcomed us with Chief Bill McLean of the Bearspaw Band.

The Stoney people have a school on the Reserve, churches, and a modern administration office where the Chiefs and Councillors sit around a triangular table so that no one is at the head but all are equal. They have a rodeo ground and a community hall. The Asian group went to the school to meet and sing for the children and their teachers, then to the Wilderness Centre – the survival school where courses are conducted each summer, three days with pack horses, three days hike etc.

The Stoneys put on a special rodeo for the *Song of Asia* group, and explained all the various events and equipment involved – the spurs and saddles, ropes and rawhide. We watched bucking broncos, calf roping, bare-back riding and bull riding. It was magnificently done. In bright sun and quite a dusty wind, I came away browner and blacker than when I arrived.

We returned to the Wilderness centre and in true outdoor style were able to wash our faces and hands in the nearby lake. One or two brave souls went swimming, but the South Pacific enthusiasm for water was almost extinguished upon discovering how close the lake was to freezing point.

Chief John Snow took us to see the Stoneys' Buffalo herd, preserved against extinction in their park. However, they do need culling from time to time and, back at the Wilderness Centre for an outdoor barbecue supper, we had buffalo roast, apple pie and ice-cream. I wrote Annejet later that I had never tasted meat I have enjoyed more – tender and of a delightful flavour.

The young Stoney men were riveted by the *Song of Asia* presentation, which went on till after midnight. At the end of the evening Chief John Snow came to the stage, wearing his head-dress of feathers, and presented *Song of Asia* with a sacred Peace Pipe, to symbolise their work of peace and reconciliation.

He invited the whole group to his home for an afternoon, an invitation which was accepted with alacrity. When we arrived we found that he had arranged for horses for any who wanted to ride, softball, badminton, horseshoe-pitching, and a barbecue of buffalo steaks in his garden.

As the sun was going down he led us through the woods behind his home, up into the mountains to his favourite spot for meditation. We walked past 'The Grand Canyon of Alberta', a breath-taking chasm with an enormous waterfall, which we came upon suddenly in the heart of the woods.

On the hilltop he made a small fire, and we sat in a circle around it, quietly thinking, listening and talking under the young pine and birch trees, the mountains high all around us. In the Indian tradition, anyone who wanted to speak got up from the circle, put a piece of wood on the fire and then said whatever they wanted, from their hearts.

I am a son of Alberta myself. Yet I experienced that evening an aspect of my country I had never known – as an old world and a new world met in brotherhood in a natural cathedral.

'It has been our tradition for many centuries,' Chief John Snow told us, 'to hear legends by the camp-fire sitting in a circle as we are now. Our elders used to teach stories of heroes of our people, reminding us of the Creator, the Great Spirit. Our people used to go to the mountain-tops, like this, to pray and get a vision, and to spend many days alone. On the mountain tops they were very close to nature and could hear the animals, birds, the voices of nature. That waterfall reminds us of the great Creator who made it, and all this beautiful creation.

'Tonight I thought we would get together, share our thoughts and experiences and perhaps the still small voice has spoken to us. If you want to speak here tonight, bring a piece of wood to the fire and then speak.

'My purpose in inviting you here is to re-strengthen your faith so you can take more courage, more strength to go with you and continue your work as you speak to the various groups. I hope tonight you have time to be reminded of the great Creator. We must live in harmony with nature and in accordance with the creation of the Great Spirit.

'I believe the fire of our traditional Indian religion has almost gone out. But within the last few years it has been re-kindled, and it is beginning to burn again. Perhaps God has given us these Reserves so we can retain our way of life, our belief, our traditions, separate from many of the non-Indians that came to this part of the world. Perhaps the time has come when we should remind many people that life is more than just trying to acquire money, buildings, material possessions, luxury. There's human life, with human values, and that life is precious. Life is a gift from God and with life God has also given us talents, many talents, and our talents vary. Some are given in music, or writing, some are in other areas. But we must use that talent to convey the message, to tell others about the great Creator and that we must live in harmony with his creation.

'You came here and gave us the chance to welcome you. You helped us re-kindle that fire which almost went out. It is burning good now, and you have added more wood to burn so that we Native people here can take courage to return to the faith of our fathers – belief in the Great Spirit.

'Thank you for coming to our country of Canada, and I pray God that he will continue to go with you and give you his strength, courage and wisdom to tell others that there is a life worth living. May the Great Spirit continue to be with you.'

Many others spoke that evening. Chief David Crowchild told how he first met Frank Buchman, how he sat and talked with him and Walking Buffalo at Mackinac, and then how, together with his wife Daisy, he travelled the world. He told us how once he had been in South Africa, in Soweto, visiting the home of a leader of the black people. Outside the little house was a throng of curious folk wanting to see a real-life 'Red Indian' in his full regalia.

'I lost quite a few pieces of my buckskin fringes to the souvenir hunters!' he told us, with a twinkle in his eye.

'When I first met MRA and my boys told me about the four absolute standards, I didn't like it. I would sometimes walk out of the room. Then I went to a conference at Mackinac with Walking Buffalo, and we met people there who treated us like kings. I have been with MRA since '58 and I am not giving up. My boys are fighting for what is right, and I stand behind them. I back them up . . . All you young people, you keep going – do not give up. There are going to be hard times, temptations, and the devil will try to hurt you and get you mad. But do not give up.'

His son Arnold put some wood on the fire. 'Commitment is like this fire,' he said. 'Every now and then you have to put wood on or the fire goes out. I need to be sure to feed the fire often enough.'

Another day we returned to the Sarcee Reserve, as official guests of the Chief and Band Council, and the Asian group were shown around the Administration offices, and spent a memorable evening in the Sarcee Bullhead Community Hall. At supper many of the Sarcee people came to eat with us, and then followed a full evening of entertainment by the Sarcee Broken Knife singing and dancing group – including the grass dance, the owl dance, in which some of the Asians were invited to join, and the spectacular chicken dance. The *Song of Asia* cast responded with an hour and a half of songs, speaking and scenes from the show, and – as always – people stayed talking for a long time afterwards. The cast invited any young Indian men and women who would care to, to travel with them across Canada and even to the Pacific, and one or two agreed with eagerness – Lee and Pearl Crowchild and Peter Manywounds among them.

After the presentation the two Crane brothers, Edwin and Leonard, spoke together from the stage to the *Song of Asia* cast and the young Sarcee people. Edwin said, 'I need change every day of my life. MRA made me look at my faith and it says "Love thy neighbour". The white man may be my neighbour. My people suffer drunkenness, greed, broken marriages – we can go down the line and name them all. But the Great Spirit can change all these things.'

Leonard said, 'I was bitter in my heart against the whites, and I went to liquor. I enjoyed getting drunk, but I ended up in jail. My parents gave me the choice, because of my drinking when I was a young man, of going to jail or of going to Mackinac Island. I figured I might be able to take a bottle with me to Mackinac Island, so I said I'd go there! Actually, the drinking stopped.

'MRA is like taking a deep breath of fresh air – cool, clean. I ask you to give this idea a bit of a chance. Absolute honesty – have I been honest with my business, with Indian Affairs? Get the dirty thinking out and start putting God's mind in. Absolute unselfishness – we all want to be in front, climbing everything for our career. Putting right what is wrong is what it is all about. Absolute love – how to love people who have done me wrong. Do you know about the guy who had the thought to return the rope he had taken from his neighbour? The neighbour thanked him, and then said, "Oh, but there was a cow at the other end of the rope – where is it?" MRA has taught me a true sense of Christianity. When you find MRA you find the spirit of the living God.'

Arnold added, 'Religion gives you a glass of clear water. MRA makes you drink it.'

Then the group went further afield, to the Blackfoot Reserve, at Gleichen, 65 miles east of Calgary, where the cast met with the Chief and Council. The Blackfoot are the largest tribe in the area, related to the Blood and Piegan peoples, with whom they formed the feared Blackfoot Confederacy.

In 1754, the Asians were told, the first white men arrived in Western Canada. In the 1850s smallpox decimated the Blackfoot people by about a third, and yet something in their traditional way of life held them together. The white man was slowly wiping out their traditional source of food – the buffalo. To the white man it was a source of money for its hide. The Blackfoot faced gradual starvation, and followed the dwindling herds as best they could. In the 1870s they gave up their territories in exchange for Reserves – a forced settlement which meant they lost their freedom to roam the country.

Regena Crowchild, Arnold's wife, comes from the Blood Reserve, 145 miles south of Calgary at Cardston, and only 17 miles from the US border. It is lovely rolling farm and ranch country near the Rockies, and is the largest Reserve in Canada, marked by very fine economic development.

The group were received by Chief Jim Shot Both Sides and Acting Chief John Chief Moon in the Council administration building, driven through the town of Cardston, the other side of the tracks from the Reserve, and then to see some of the activities on the Reserve. They have a factory there, producing prefabricated wooden buildings which are sold all across Canada, and in Montana also. They also produce the foremost Canadian Indian newspaper, on modern computerised equipment. The names of the Blood people tell a story of their own – Chief Jim Shot Both Sides, Chief John Chief Moon, Councillor Ben Scout, Councillor Pete Standing Alone, Councillor Frank Eagle Tailfeathers, Yvonne Shouting.

We drove for an hour across dusty track roads to the Band Ranches, where a small rodeo display was specially staged, including trying to break in a really wild horse, which got the better of three or four cowboys. In the evening the Asians were again entertained by Indian dancing, and responded with songs and scenes from *Song of Asia*.

Our hosts thought of every detail and spared no effort to care for and get to know each one. I was asked to speak in the community hall of the Blood Reserve, at the end of the evening presentation, and said, 'I stand here a different man than when I arrived, because you have made me, as an Albertan, very proud of what you have done here. I would like to see the whole world know about it. I believe it is but a preparation for what the people of this area are meant to initiate for our country, for the American continent, and out to the world.'

This was a particularly significant time, because two days earlier on the nearby Piegan reserve, Nelson Small Legs Jr, a young man of 23, son of Cllr Nelson Small Legs Sr who had been part of the invitation committee for *Song of Asia* to Canada, was found dead of gunshot wounds. He was a director of the American Indian Movement in Canada, married, with two young children. AIM has been known as an extreme, often violent, movement, but Nelson Jr had himself been opposed to the use of violence unless absolutely necessary. By his body were found letters seeming to indicate that he had taken his life, in protest against the way his people were being treated by the Federal Government.

A fortnight before his death, Nelson Small Legs Jr had spent a morning with the young Asians, speaking to them about his work and his beliefs, and answering questions.

'I am not a terrorist,' he told the group. 'I do not know how to use an automatic weapon. I do not know the martial arts or hand-to-hand combat. The only weapon I have as a Native American is truth. Nobody can beat truth.

'Here in Canada we don't advocate violence, with AIM. I don't say "Burn buildings in the name of the people back home." I cannot do that, it would be hurting myself. If two buffalo fight, the prairie grass gets torn up. The people who suffer are the grass-roots people – they will suffer and have nothing. 'Today AIM is a warrior society and the people that met you at Calgary Airport are our leaders and elders. AIM is composed of men and women who want social change. We may not be able to go back to buffalo days, but we can deepen our spiritual ways today. The Peace Pipe is an ordinary pipe – the bowl is made out of stone, the stem of wood. The stone represents the earth, and what you smoke is given you by the sun. You don't worship the sun. It is the Great Spirit you worship. We have survived here 45,000 years living in harmony with nature.

'Patience is the essence of everything. If you have patience you can take it anywhere you like. It may take all your life. We may have every justification to take up the gun and to walk down to the Parliament Buildings and blow heads off.

That is not going to solve anything. There are right roads to take.

'With white people we can work together to save Canada, the North American continent and the world. I am not a racist. I do not hate the white people nor the dominating society, but I speak the truth about it. I am able to work with people.'

Nelson Small Legs Jr had been at one or two *Song of Asia* events and meetings after that. Only two days before his death, he had arrived at 10.30 at night, wanting to talk and share experiences with each one of them, and was full of plans for the future, including a visit by them to the Piegan Reserve where he lived. So the news of his death came as a great shock to all. I and some others went to visit his family the next day.

I wrote Annejet in London:

Arnold sees our presentation on the Reserves as God-timed. We see the living evidence of a world force offering an alternative way to frustration and violence. At Piegan we called on Chief Nelson Small Legs and his wife, and the young widow of Nelson Jr. Niketu Iralu gave the family his prized Naga shawl, which was then draped over the coffin. The family were much moved. The tragedy has been national news. AIM interprets the death as the signal for 'all-out war' on the Indian Affairs bureaucracy.

The event has focussed for us all how genuine our touch with people needs to be. That is the issue in almost every nation today. The Director of the Calgary Indian Affairs Office told us he fears demonstrations and violence following the funeral.

Nelson Jr's younger brother was on the radio news, in an interview talking of the death, and referred to the note found by Nelson Jr's body, saying that he and his people were going to declare war on the government. But Nelson Small Legs Sr was on national TV, asking the young Indians to think how to work for their aims without violence, for violence was not the way of his son.

In particular one performance of a scene from *Song of*

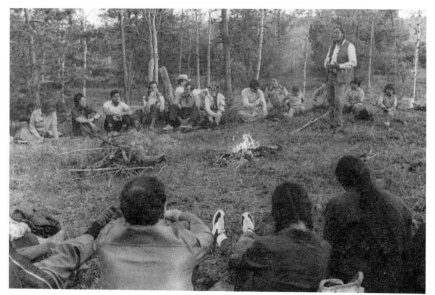

Chief John Snow speaking to the *Song of Asia* group at a camp-fire evening he arranged on the Stoney Reserve.

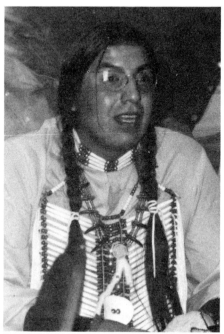

Nelson Small Legs Jr told the *Song of Asia* group, 'The only weapon I have as a Native American is truth.'

Asia, given that memorable night on the Blood Reserve, was like an electric current. The atmosphere was uncertain – many young men wanted blood revenge for the death of Nelson Jr. This scene, a true story from the North-East of India, told of a family in which two sons went to fight in a guerilla war, and lost their lives; it showed the anguish of the third son and of their mother. Should he, too, go and take up arms and attempt to avenge his brothers? Or could he be the one to break the chain of hate, and make peace with his enemies, for the sake of the living?

In that small hall, with no stage lighting, scenery, wings, few costumes, I have never seen that scene done more grippingly or movingly – the answer to hatred, bitterness and revenge.

Chief David Crowchild said of that moment, 'It really affected the people. A lot of people took it very seriously, the play, and I think a lot of people changed in that way.'

The *Song of Asia* group moved north to fulfil pre-arranged engagements in and around Edmonton, and I was delighted to be able to take them to Vegreville for a day's visit. The 35 members of the cast were received by the Mayor and some of his councillors. The town where I was born is a small and friendly place with a predominantly Ukrainian population, and is known throughout the whole of Canada as the city of the million dollar Easter egg. The Egg, made of aluminum triangles, was erected to commemorate the centenary of the RCMP. It displays a significant Ukrainian religious design, accented by a mosaic of brilliant colours.

I wrote Annejet about the day, which meant a great deal to me personally.

May 23rd, '76, Edmonton
Yesterday at Vegreville was a marvel. We were welcomed by the Mayor at a restaurant and given a marvellous tea. I got Muriel Patterson (my former teacher) and her two sisters to come. The officials of the Lions Club did all the organising. The Mayor told us about the Egg. I replied saying the Almighty must want something really big to be hatched from so giant an egg – perhaps a quality

of home and civic life based on what is right not who is right.

We had a most moving time at the cemetery, where my parents and little sister are buried. I used the occasion to share the deepest things with the Mayor and those with him. The bus driver wept! I was grateful to be able to include my friends in a very deep and treasured part of my life and experience. As we left, it was suddenly decided by our hosts that we must stay for a barbecue in the park at 6 pm, which we did.

We were certainly God-led in our timing to be on the Reserves, establishing the fact that there is an alternative to violence and frustration. Roy Littlechief has persuaded his AIM colleagues to have a go at talking with Government people, both provincial and federal, before taking violent action.

Nelson Small Legs Sr is a big man in every sense of the word. He stands well over six feet, and in his Piegan regalia he has the presence and dignity typical of his people. One morning he told the young Asian men and women about his life.

'For many years we lived in a one-room log cabin. My son spent the first five years of his life there. I worked on the oil rigs up north, on the heavy equipment. I worked in Edmonton and BC. Though I have an artificial right eye, I used to drive heavy trucks all over the Province. One weekend I came home to see my boys and suddenly it hit me – a heart attack. I had to learn to walk all over again. The doctor gave me pills and told me I would have to take them for the rest of my life. It was like the end of the world for me. I started drinking, but after two years I quit it. My wife has stuck by me in this.

'I went into politics on my Reserve, and then it hit me again – another heart attack. I was in that hospital for two weeks. The doctors told me when I came out that I must never drive alone again. I was not afraid, because I knew that the Great Spirit was there. I used to drive a grader on the roads on my Reserve, but after my time in hospital I could not do that any more. I decided to return to my Indian traditions and customs. I wanted to ride in the Calgary Stampede, but I had no outfit, only a horse! So someone lent me buckskins.

'I wanted to help my fellow Indians who had problems with alcohol and drugs, and to get them back on their feet when they had been in trouble. I had been told not to drive alone, but I knew I must help my people. The week after I got out of that hospital I drove alone to a meeting in Banff, and there I met a lady who offered me a job, working to help my people. I took it.

'Since then I have driven thousands of miles in my car, and my truck, helping my people. If my heart is going to stop it will happen – I don't have to sit and wait for it. And if it does happen, I am training other people to carry on the work. That Person up there is the best friend I have got.'

Song of Asia was invited to attend a dinner in the Parliament buildings in Ottawa, together with their hosts, the Chiefs of Treaty #7. The evening was hosted by Senators and leading parliamentarians. The Minister for Indian Affairs, the Hon Judd Buchanan, 10 Senators and 26 MPs were also present.

After dinner and a brief presentation by the *Song of Asia* group, Chief Bill McLean of the Stoneys said, 'I feel if the Canadian Government could only understand us at grass-roots level, both sides could find a solution.'

Senator Paul Yuzyk, one of the sponsors of the occasion responded. He assured the Chiefs that the parliamentarians present would co-operate in solving their problems through 'consultation rather than confrontation'.

Nelson Small Legs Sr later told us of his meeting at that dinner with the Minister of Indian Affairs – the man whose attitude had focussed Nelson Jr's protests.

'Buchanan sat by me, shook hands with me. And I told him, "I have no personal feelings against you and your family", and we shook on that. After a while he asked me for a second time, "What can I do?" What could I tell him? Will I tell him "Give me back my son?" I was bitter in the first place, but today I'm not. "I am inviting *Song of Asia* to come to Piegan Reserve to help our people," I told him.'

Senator Ches Carter from Newfoundland, who co-sponsored the dinner, said later, 'The Asian group is certainly God's gift to Canada at this crucial point in our history, which could very well determine whether Canada will continue to exist as a nation or split apart into a number of self-centred states. It is particularly encouraging to learn of the new relationships that have developed between the Indians and the Hon Judd Buchanan and the officials of his Department.'

Later in July we again met the Lt Governor of Alberta, the Hon Ralph Steinhauer. When we reported to him on our time in Ottawa, he replied, 'Nelson Small Legs Sr could have tipped the balance in either direction after the death of his son. This is a very crucial time for our people in this country. I am glad Nelson is doing what he is doing today.'

Chapter Eighteen

ALL IN THE SAME CANOE

THE *SONG OF ASIA* group moved on to Québec, led by Chief David Crowchild, Daisy his wife, and others from Alberta.

Kahnawake Reserve, on the outskirts of Montréal is the home of about 5,000 Iroquois people, making it the second most populous reserve in Canada. The people are also known as Mohawk Indians, and are famous for their courage and skill. They are originally a river people, pilots to the fur traders' canoes, but lost their shoreline when the St Lawrence Seaway was built. They have always responded to a challenge – and today are well-known as fearless steel workers, precariously earning their living high above the New York streets, and out west on the Golden Gate Bridge.

Representatives of four Native tribes, two from Eastern Canada and two from Western Canada, led *Song of Asia* onto the stage officially to open the Kahnawake Indian days. Chief Andrew Delisle of the Iroquois was President of the Indians of Québec Association, and Chief Mike McKenzie of the Algonquin of Kipawa, in NW Québec, had driven 360 miles with his wife to be present.

Chief Ron Kirby of Kahnawake, spoke at the end of the evening. 'Material answers are not the solution I am looking for, for my people. I think tonight I have found something that is the solution.'

At Trois-Rivières, the Asians met for an evening of discussion with a group of young people, former drug addicts. After a time of meditation, one young man of the local group said, 'I noticed you write down your thoughts – I think it is a good idea, because sometimes you forget what you think, and also, by writing them down, you can use them later.'

A Catholic priest said, 'The idea of reflection and writing down your thoughts is a good one. I'm surprised I didn't think of it before. If we all did it, we would have something to say at our meetings, because we could share our experiences.' I was glad to have the chance, in Trois-Rivières, to spell out my vision and beliefs about Canada:

'I want to say one thing, as an English Canadian. Out in the West, in Alberta, if you have English blood, for some reason you think if there's anything going on you ought to be running it. Also you think, if there is any difference of opinion, that you're more apt to be right than the other fellow. Well, then I married a Dutch girl. And she told me just exactly how I was behaving. She changed me. And I began to get a more realistic understanding of myself and of my people. But with that came a growing respect and evaluation of the other people who were not English – the Ukrainians who formed the majority of the population in the town where I was born, the Native peoples, and the glorious people of French Canada.

'My apology to all those people is to dedicate the rest of my life to bring about this change and this spirit to my country, the United States, Europe, Africa and Asia.'

Chief David Crowchild said of the time in the Province of Québec, 'A lot of people seem to have been woken up by Song of Asia, even white people, like those in Trois-Rivières. I always opened the presentation with a prayer, sometimes I used my language, sometimes I used the Lord's Prayer. It seemed to affect the people, they'd think we came on the warpath or something!'

Shortly after the first Song of Asia performance in Kahnawake, Chief Andrew Delisle was elected to replace Chief Ron Kirby, and he invited the whole cast of Song of Asia to return to Kahnawake. On this second visit the travelling group stayed in homes on the Reserve for three or four days. Huron Chief Max Gros-Louis, an executive member of the Indians of Québec Association, introduced the French première of Chant de l'Asie (Song of Asia) to a cosmopolitan Montréal audience.

Chief Aurelien Gill, from the Pointe Bleue Montagnais (Algonquin) Reserve in the north of Québec, said, 'We Indians and you from the Third World have a lot in common with our traditions and values, but at this point we are losing them. We need to return to them and then share them with the rest of the world.'

After presenting a Bamboo dance from his country as part of the evening's performance, a young man from the Muslim minority in the Philippines said, 'I am aware of the ill-feeling and resentment between the English and French speaking people. I am very interested to see how you resolve this issue. The answer you will find will affect our countries.'

Diane Paré, a Québecoise, replied, 'Yes, in Canada we French are a minority, and we accuse the English of treating us badly. But for the Native people, we are all palefaces. I feel I am also to be blamed for the exploitation and indifference we have had towards the Native people. We wanted so much to get them integrated into our society that they have lost almost all of their culture. I ask forgiveness from the Chiefs here today.'

One of the audience said after the presentation, 'Tonight as I sat and watched the show, I felt all my hate and aggression towards other people melt.'

A young woman from Laos spoke in French at a public performance *Chant de l'Asie* in Montréal. Rothay Chantharasy, speaking after performing a Lao flower dance with her sister Ramphay, told the audience, 'We are now refugees. There are millions homeless like us. We come from a large family, which sometimes has its difficulties. But as a family we have learned to forgive and to ask for forgiveness. And most of all we try to listen to and obey the inner voice which speaks in every heart. That's what unites us.

'Our country lost its freedom because we did not find the answer to materialism and the corruption in left and in right. To create freedom and peace we have to sacrifice our prejudices, our bad feelings, our jealousies.'

John Bocock, Albertan dairy farmer, said, 'I'm convinced that more important than who you are or where you come from is what you've decided to do to put right the things that are wrong.' He spoke of the ambitions that had led his family to rent more land, increasing the size of their farm until it was larger than they could farm properly. They had conviction to give up their rented land. 'It means that we can produce more per acre because we can take better care of our land, and it also means we don't have to work 16 hours a day – and we can even get away on occasion to join our friends, as I am doing now!'

Financially, the size and scope of the *Song of Asia* campaign was an immense challenge, running into many thousands of dollars. People responded marvellously to it, by offering hospitality, meals, transport, and contributing in hard cash an amount equivalent to the entire MRA Canada budget for the previous year.

A grant from the Alberta Government Department of Culture enabled the group to accept the Chiefs' invitation to return to Alberta from Québec, in particular for the visit to the Piegan Reserve which had been postponed earlier, and for a conference in Calgary.

This conference was conceived especially for those who had come in contact on the earlier visit of the Asian group, and who had expressed interest.

(P to A)
August 5th, '76, Calgary
We have had 200 at the conference. A most amazing turn-out of Indian leadership, including Ernest Tootoosis, almost legendary Medicine Man from Saskatchewan; Chief Si Baker from Vancouver who wants the group to visit his Reserve; Kitpow, a Medicine Man from near Kelowna, graduate of Eton and Oxford! . . . . . Last night it ended with a pow-wow. We had a wonderful hoop dance and chicken dance.

I was called up at one point, and David Crowchild, in full regalia, gave me an Indian name, with beaded moccasins and gloves to mark the occasion. The name is 'Thunder Child' – 'Cha Mayza' in the Sarcee language. As part of the ceremony Chief David gave me the traditional shove on the shoulder. It was nearly strong enough to topple me over!

One AIM man, Alvin Wolf Leg, said, 'In the absolute standards is the ultimate weapon for the Indian advance.'

Pearl Crowchild, who had been travelling with the *Song of Asia* group, spoke at a conference session, alongside her father, Chief Gordon. 'I was going to prove to the white man that Indians are just as good as whites,' she said. 'I became very bitter towards them. Then *Song of Asia* came to Canada. I met them at the airport, but I wasn't going to change my ways. It took me two letters and two talks with my parents to become completely honest with them about myself. I had difficulty in deciding to join *Song of Asia* because my friends didn't agree with it and wanted me to stay home. I guess I just wanted to prove that I could do something useful with my life, and I think I've found the answer.'

Laurent Gagnon, one of the men responsible for the programme of MRA in Canada, spoke of his home Province of Québec. 'Our worst sin is always blaming the English speakers and everybody else,' he said. 'We want them to understand us and change completely before we stop pushing them to be different.

'We wish to be loved by them, but we lack patience and are often not very lovable. Furthermore, it is clear that both of us, French and English Canadians, are in the same canoe vis-à-vis the Native people and have a common sin towards them.

'The underdog feeling can blind minorities in the same way that arrogance on the part of the majority can provoke the worst in those who feel badly treated. The feelings of people have to be taken as seriously as facts of history. We still all have a lot to learn.'

In amongst the thousands of square miles of some of the most beautiful prairie lands lies the Piegan Reservation. At the invitation of Cllr Nelson Small Legs Sr and his family, the cast of *Song of Asia* took part in the annual Piegan Indian days, and gave their presentation to an audience of 300 in the Crow Lodge complex. To have the cast living in the homes of families on the Reserve, and also in Pincher Creek, a small town eight miles away, gave impetus to the creation of a new relationship between the two communities.

Nelson Small Legs introduced the stage presentation to his people saying, 'This play opened my eyes.'

Among the audience were the Hon Bob Bogle, Minister without Portfolio, responsible for Native Affairs for the Province of Alberta, and some of his fellow MLAs. Speaking

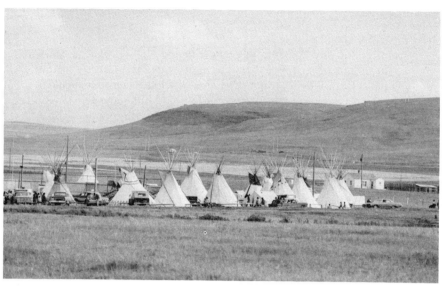

Teepees at the annual Piegan Indian days, in amongst some of the most beautiful prairie lands of Southern Alberta.

'At the pow-wow at the end of the Calgary conference in 1976, Chief David Crowchild gave me the name "Thunder Child". His traditional shove on the shoulder was nearly strong enough to topple me over?'

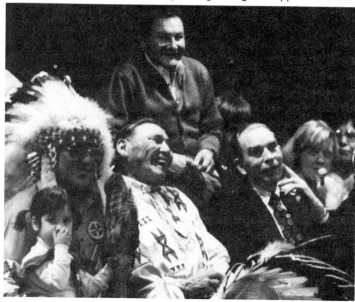

after the show, Mr Bogle said, 'When I first saw this show in Edmonton, I was moved in a way I had not thought possible. I was so touched that when I stood up to speak to the audience at the end, I forgot I was a politician. The reason I asked my colleagues to come along with me tonight is because the message you have to share with us, the message of co-operation and working together, is one that needs to be heard on both sides. And together we can succeed.'

After this the group moved to the beautiful country on the West coast, to British Columbia, where they gave their presentation in the Long House on the Squamish Reserve in Vancouver, and also on Vancouver Island. No one who was present will ever forget the salmon bake we were given there.

Rakai Tomoana, a Maori, told us of a decision she had taken two years earlier. It was, she said, 'to live without the two sources I thought did the most harm to my people – God and the white man.

'I had a picture of the kind of world I wanted to see, but because the quality of my own life was so low, it was impossible for me to be effective in any way.

'Three months ago I made another decision – to take one hour each day to listen to God and to let him completely direct my life, and to live the four absolute standards of honesty, purity, unselfishness and love. It hasn't been easy and I don't envisage it to be easy, but because of this decision I have now learned that I can live alongside the Europeans, accept with gratitude the good they have done my people, and fight for them to be different where I see injustice.

'I have also learned the responsibility of being a Maori, a minority, to be responsible for the future of my people and my children, and not be weighted down and obsessed with blame for the past.'

We made the beautiful ferry trip over to Vancouver Island, and drove to the reserves of the Seshaht and Opetchesaht at Port Alberni. *Song of Asia* presentations were given there, and in Victoria, and the group were generously welcomed by the local people.

Verna McDougall, daughter of Cllr Wilf McDougall of the Piegan Band, and grand-daughter of the Band's Chief, joined the Asian group for some weeks shortly before the young Asians dispersed to return to their own countries, and she spoke at the end of one presentation, 'The reason I'm here is I have a feeling that our people need to accept something that will change all the bitterness that they have inside them. I think that the next generation has to take its stand.'

Wilf McDougall, Councillor of the Piegan Band, told of one of his experiences with *Song of Asia*. 'You know, this has really done something to myself and my family. We seem to have come together. I myself used to drink a lot, but I'm moving away from liquor now. My wife was present at the wedding of two of your company, and she told me, "Wilf, there was no liquor and you know what? We had more fun at the wedding than any other wedding I've been to." This is a lesson – if you stop and think about it. It's a lesson. Usually at a wedding, the first thing that comes out is a bottle.'

Lee Crowchild, son of Chief Gordon Crowchild, says of his people, 'Unfortunately my generation among Indian people have begun to lose the values we had before. To get through problems of assimilation, and so on, we have to get back to those moral values, and the tribes must get back to the source of inspiration which was theirs since time began.'

Following the Song of Asia visit to Canada, the Chiefs of Treaty #7 received an invitation from the Maori Elders of the Takitimu Canoe to go to New Zealand.

In January 1977 Arnold Crowchild, with Chief Leo Pretty Young Man of the Blackfoot, Chief Bill McLean, Chief Simon Baker, elder of the Squamish people of the West Coast, and over 50 Native peoples travelled to New Zealand. Their trip was conceived as part of the Treaty #7 Centennial celebrations.

Chief Leo Pretty Young Man talked about his experiences some weeks later:

'We went to New Zealand, quite a few of us went down there to this conference. 29-30 nations were represented, and we spoke, we went to the maraes – the Maori meeting places – and with the experiences I went through down there, I came back to my people, and I was asked immediately to go on TV.

'I did it. This is amazing – I spoke with representatives from the CBC TV crew, and they asked a lot of questions –

"Why did you say this or that?"; "Why did you do it?" I simply answered that this is something which is needed. Nine of them in the room, and I told them, "Why don't you take one minute, and ask the guy inside you – who am I?". These nine people left without answering me or anything, though a month or two later I started receiving apologies from them.

'That same day I received a phone call about 4.00 from my town council who called a meeting that evening at 7.30, a joint meeting, something which never happened before. The reserve and the town of Gleichan is divided by the rail-track, and we've not worked too well together. I was surprised. So I jumped in my car and went down to the meeting, and since that day we have had a monthly meeting. It was because of the TV interview about my visit to NZ.'

Arnold Crowchild said to me that the presence in Canada of *Song of Asia* was living evidence of an alternative way for the Canadian people.

Chapter Nineteen

CAPE TOWN TO CALGARY

IN OCTOBER 1977 I was invited by friends to South Africa
– my first visit.

(P to A)
October 6th, '77 flying between Nairobi and Jo'burg,
just passing Salisbury

I slept fitfully – read quite a bit. A very good talk with
a young NY investment broker who with his wife is going
on safari in Kenya. I had a bit of a headache due to the
poor position of my neck while I tried to sleep. But my
talk with this man quickly dispelled all aches and pains!

October 8th, '77 Jo'burg

This is a fascinating country and a fiery crucible. What
has struck me so far is the deafness. People don't hear
each other's words or anguish. Blaming others, blacks,
whites, coloured, ideologies, the English, the Afrikaaners,
has conditioned much thinking. And blame creates colossal apathy.

. . . It seems to me South Africa is focussing a crucial
issue. Will the Christians and people of faith demonstrate
to the world that we are the greatest and swiftest force
for change in the world – a revolution where everyone
wins and no one loses.

Christianity is judged in the world by our public performance and policies, not only by our private devotions.
This country gives hope and underlines the way forward.
If we transcend wrong racial attitudes here, our civilization will live, if not it will die. The flow of history can
be turned from here.

It is clear that those who put the blame on somebody
else become blind and apathetic to where they themselves
have been wrong and can do differently. And this apathy

195

feeds frustration; then violence of one sort or another is employed in an effort to get the attention of the other group.

Change is needed. I think it little matters who begins. It should be easier for those to begin who are only 1% wrong, than for those who are 99% wrong. You see many promising characters narrowed and desiccated by the bitterness that comes from hurt feelings – but too proud to make amends and to start afresh. I guess most of us shrink from pain – and from those who produce it. The way one gives wide berth to a horse who has once planted his hoof in your stomach! But an openness to pain, without bitterness, becomes a healing force and a redeeming power.

I heard today of a 12 year old black boy who used to steal and came 46th out of 47 in his class. Last Christmas he decided to live by listening to the voice of Truth in his heart – he stopped stealing and became sixth in his class.

October 11th, '77

The spokesman for the 'committee of 10' in Soweto spent the evening with us. This committee is begging the Government to let the people themselves tackle education, the housing (often there are 10-20 people to a room), the unemployment, the transportation (also overcrowded, with a lot of crime), and a rising incidence of malnutrition.

20 years ago a Bantu Education Board was set up for the blacks. Where a white student has 660 units of money allocated for his training, the Bantu Board can grant only 37.5 units! The quality of teaching is poor, schools have no science laboratories, recently a lower primary school in a white middle-class area was built at a cost of two-and-a-half million rand; 42 black schools were allotted half that amount for building costs. Joey Daneel [the wife of a Dutch Reformed Minister and former Springbok rugby player, who had known and worked with Buchman] spoke on Monday morning from the heart as an Afrikaaner. She was talking of the callousness of Kruger when he said on TV of Biko's death, 'It leaves me cold.'

'Just to say sorry doesn't mean anything,' she said, 'God

forgive us – nothing else can help us. We may not be able to take on the sins of our fathers, but we can take on the sins of our group and decide to try to restore for them.'

October 17th, '77

I went with friends to the Kruger National Park and saw a huge elephant beside the road eating grass and stripping trees of their leaves. Impala, a beautiful deer, by the hundreds. 16 giraffe together nibbling leaves off trees, families of baboons – some with the young upside down clinging to their stomachs as they walked, black-faced monkeys by the score. Four hippo yawning and luxuriating, blowing and snorting in a pool. Some monkeys, if you stop, jump on the car and ride with you till you stop again. I saw a hyena and jackals, a sable antelope with black front and noble antlers, warthogs, scores of zebra, buffalo, heron, etc etc. And a secretary bird which flaps its wings at a snake to confuse it, then it picks up the snake, flies high and drops it, and lands on it as the snake hits the ground!

October 18th, '77 Jo'burg

As one wise man said, 'I know not what is in the heart of a scoundrel, but I know what is in the heart of a good man, and it is horrible!'

Here only heroic, convinced personalities without fear or bitterness can do what is needed. There is no substitute for lives being transformed.

October 29th, '77, Capetown

We had nine holes of golf on the Royal Cape Club course! I played quite well – getting a par and a birdie on the last two holes to even the score!

In 1899 when there was the Gold Rush the Big Powers began dictating, 'give votes to the immigrants.' The Africans replied, 'You don't want the vote, you want our country'. Holland, England and France have all had their attempts to dominate.

Blacks and whites move in closed circuits – separately – so the people of real dedication on each side don't know each other. This is a significant role MRA plays here, making such encounters possible.

The squatter areas are being cleared by bulldozer, people have temporary homes in churches etc. Said one woman to the man in charge of bulldozing, 'Are you a Christian?' 'Yes,' he replied. Then she asked, 'Is this the work of God?' He was confused and embarrassed. Said one old squatter, at a hearing in the city hall, 'O God forgive me, if I have done anything to deserve this.' People wept.

Society here is highly organized. And everything stems from the church. The easiest way to be pushed out of the establishment is to belong to something like MRA, for it is interpreted as moving away from the church.

It makes you think through Christ's truth in a situation like this – treat others the way you wish to be treated, or you brutalise yourself and your society, the sure road to chaos and control. Seek first God's rule in people's lives, and all else will be added. Unless people are changing all we do is irrelevant. We will be on the side-lines, and in the back eddies of history. Bashing the whites to gain favour with the blacks will not do. This continent needs more than sanctions from America. It needs Penn's and Washington's love of the truth and hate of the lie.

November 2nd, '77, Pretoria
This experience here for me means a purifying of my dedication to God and his will – to make the whole of life and living dependent on Christ – a great consciousness of the need to be obedient. For God alone can do what needs to be done here – and I believe he longs to do it – and is hindered only by the holdbacks and compromises in placing all of life for the doing of his will.

I made various transatlantic trips during the next months, continuing the work already in hand both in Canada and in the United States. As usual, I kept Annejet in touch.
(P to A)
February 3rd, '77 Montréal
I have discovered a number of my (medical) class-mates

seem to be on the point of retiring! I don't see why they all retire so young!

Trudeau quotes Sir Wilfrid Laurier in a book I've been reading – 'French Canadians do not have opinions, only emotions.' This I regard more as a judgement on the English than on the French, for to our shame we used the democratic process for our own ends, and gave much reason for them to distrust their future in the hands of the Protestant Anglos.

. . . How are EA and Digna getting on at school? I hope our tobogganing didn't knock all the arithmetic out of their systems!

June 24th, '77, Montréal, Saint-Jean-Baptiste Day

Much enthusiasm here for today. Saint-Jean-Baptiste is the Patron Saint of the French Canadians, and this is Québec National Day. It began last night with a huge rally in the Olympic Stadium, with dozens of Québec French singers and performers. It has become an expression of the new French-Canadian confidence.

. . . . I had a good time with one of my younger friends from Québec, who felt I had undercut him with people in the West in March. I had not agreed with him on every point about Québec, but as I reflected I felt that was not the central issue. I think it was more that I have had a teacher-pupil relationship (so characteristic of imperialists), parent-child, boss-worker attitude, of which I was not wholly conscious, instead of realising that we all need to learn from each other. It is what the Native people feel about the rest of us. I shared this with him and others at the breakfast table next morning.

July 2nd, '77

My aim is to bring this country under God's control. To do his will in everything, as the Good Lord gives me insight and strength. The medium is the message. What we *are* speaks far more effectively than what we *say*. In this sense, true care for people begins with our own personalities, developed to their highest expression. To be 'perfect' as our Heavenly Father is perfect, means apparently to be 'full-grown', fully developed. It is what Christ does for us, when we expose ourselves fully to his influence. Then growth in freedom and power is inevitable, without struggle.

Unexpectedly, my very good friend Arnold Crowchild, aged 36, died on April 13th, 1978, after a two-week illness. He left his wife, Regena, and three daughters – Jean, June and Faith. It was a big shock to all his friends. We had worked together very closely through the last few years.

I was privileged to be asked to speak at his funeral.

(P to A)
April 18th, '78, Calgary

Yesterday's service for Arnold was a tremendous tribute. Bill Pattemore, a prominent Alberta Liberal, spoke in the Crowchild home the evening before. He said Trudeau had spoken to him, and he to Arnold, about running for parliament, for any party, as he was the type of man needed.

Nelson Small Legs spoke in the home before we left for the church, of how much Arnold had meant in his own life. A young Sarcee said, 'My, the outreach of that man's life. I am beginning to understand what he's doing'. Elders from Sarcee, the Crees in Hobbema, the Stoneys, prayed by Arnold's side in their own language. Many hymns were sung the evening before. They asked me to speak at the service. I said that Arnold's was not the life of a saint, but he was a true warrior. His perfection was not his strength, but his refusal to be blackmailed out of the fight by his failings was his strength. I made the point that when I go I do not wish to have any relationship that is unclear, and live with the same generosity of attitude to others that God has towards me.

Death is a time of participation with the family. Everybody comes to the house to sing hymns, pray, sit silently with Arnold in the room. We all returned for a feast in Arnold's home from the cemetery.

His vision for his country and mine still lives. This is how he expressed it once:

'A minority can be the conscience of a country. I have been in Québec and Northern Ireland. Governments get excited about the French Canadians or the Catholics in Northern Ireland. They don't realise that these minorities can touch their nation's conscience. And we minorities don't realise that, having touched this conscience with the authority of having been oppressed, we have something to live for and to give, to put right what is wrong in the world . . . I want to take responsibility, regardless of what anyone else does.'

Chapter Twenty

A SENSE OF DIRECTION

SEVERAL YEARS AGO, 'Believe It Or Not' was a regular feature in some Canadian newspapers. The cartoonist would illustrate the story. One such column told of one of my Dad's brothers, who was sailing in the Bay of Biscay and tossed a block of wood over the side, with his name on it. A few months later this wooden block washed up on the water's edge of the harbour in Canna, at the foot of the path leading to the house where he was born, and where his parents were still living – believe it or not.

In 1978 we took our daughters on a family visit to Canna, and stayed on the Island three days. We were given hospitality in the home of friends where an aunt of mine had lived. The family refused to take any recompense. The son of the home was a lobster fisherman. Sadly a year later he was drowned in a storm. The mother of the house provided our girls with a bottle, in which they put a piece of paper with their names and address, and then, after consulting the ferry captain, they threw it over the side of the boat at the place where he indicated. Two months later they received a letter from a couple who had found the bottle on the shores of Skye and had the goodness of heart to write.

God has given us a marvellously rich family relationship – and I cherish it. Having two daughters has brought a wonderful new dimension to life.

Edith Anne is very proud of her Canadian passport – even though she was born in Holland, we applied for Canadian citizenship for her. Yet from her education in London and Oxford she feels very English.

Digna I think grew up feeling thoroughly English and has a British passport – though of course both girls are a bit Dutch as well, and used to love our family holidays at Annejet's parents' cottage on the lakes in the north of Holland. I believe we have managed to go there every summer since the girls were born.

Edith Anne studied English and French Literature at the Oxford Poly. She sometimes used to bring her friends in to talk with us when they had problems. She went to Aix-en-Provence in her second year, and for her spring break she and I went to Morocco together - a wonderful chance for me to renew some of the friendships made when I first was there with Buchman in the '50s. Digna and Annejet were in Dulwich.

We received a heart-warming reception from our old friends, Ahmed and Malika Guessous and Pierre and Jeanine Chavanne. And I was very glad to meet Abdessadeq El Glaoui again, the son of El Glaoui, who had been instrumental in the change of attitude that took place in his father.

Edith Anne was a stalwart in translation, as I do not speak French very well. And the men of the party were able to get in a few holes of golf on the Casablanca course, which rejoiced me greatly.

(P to A)
February 24th, '84, Casablanca

What a remarkable daughter and daughters we have. EA has won everyone – with her gentleness and disposition. She shared with a nurse (a friend of Jeanine Chavanne) in Marrakech the other day, 'I'm going to work with MRA out of gratitude for what God has done for me.' You see here the real unity of heart and mind of all those – whether Muslim or Christian – who put God first. To me this is one reason why Frank Buchman and this work were raised up. Where theology (ideas in the brain) divides, ideology (the way we live and care for people) unites.

Edith Anne went on to get 1st class Honours in English and French Literature and Language – in spite of quite severe headaches as a result of having glandular fever when she was 15. Then she had a year at drama school in Guildford.

She has a real gift for showing emotion on the stage, and loves acting because she can really let go on the stage. More than once she has had us in tears in the front row. She had several parts in plays at Oxford, and also in Caux during the summer conferences.

Digna, like her mother, is very artistic. They love the same sort of things – for example making clothes, or re-decorating the house. She is extremely creative.

I'm not sure how well we did as parents of teenage children. There are likely many things we could have done better. I think it is fair to say that to start with Edith Anne was rather a conformist, though none of us realised it at the time. For example, the first time we saw her in the part of a rebellious teenager on stage, it was quite an eye-opener for her parents. Why we should have been so naïve I don't know. And then once she told us how jealous she was of her sister, because she did exactly what she felt like, and didn't give a damn. She said to us, 'I know what's right in my head, but it's not in my heart. I know if I don't live a certain way, it's going to hurt people, but I don't want your advice, I'm just telling you what I feel.'

We tried very hard not to say anything, but prayed a lot. It was a year later that she came to us and said, 'It has been such a marvellous year at Oxford, and I feel God has given me so much without asking anything in return, that I feel I want to serve him because I love him and not because I have to. I want to serve him out of gratitude.' It was a watershed.

Digna has always been a completely different kettle of fish. There was one occasion when she had been talking to me, and felt I wasn't listening to her. I replied that I had heard every word she had said, and repeated the conversation back to her. Her retort was, 'Well, then you should say something, because otherwise I don't know whether you've heard me or not!'

Probably we could have been much freer with the girls, especially Digna, about our views on sex, relationships, drugs and the like, and seeking out what they themselves felt. It was naïve to assume that because we had certain views, they would have the same!

It is not easy to be a wise father. It is much easier to give your kids what they want, hoping it is going to make them happy. Sometimes I was like putty in their hands, and Annejet had to enlighten me on the deviousness of the female of the species. She often told me I was too soft, while in turn I used to believe she was too hard with the girls. So we had to turn to the Almighty for wisdom.

When Digna was 16 we tried our best to be open-hearted and open-minded about her friends, but there was one young man in particular who made it rather hard. And there were two occasions when she stayed away over night without letting us know where she was, which gave great concern to her mother and to me.

She thought school was boring, and wanted to leave without doing any 'A' levels, and become a hairdresser. Her idea was to share a flat with a girl-friend who was also training to be a hairdresser. Neither of them could really afford it, but we felt we should let her try.

They found a one-room place, with a kitchen at one end – and then decided to go and get a cat from the Battersea Dogs' Home, but instead came back with two puppies. As both of them were working all day long, you can imagine the sort of state the flat was in when they returned, even though the dogs were placed 'securely' in one corner.

Six or seven months after she had moved out Annejet and I were supposed to go to Canada again. We really wondered whether we should go, leaving Digna totally on her own – her flat had no phone, and the only hope we had of contacting her was on Sundays at lunchtime, when she might be at the home of a friend.

But we felt God's leading to us to go to Canada, and asking us to trust Digna to him.

One day in Ottawa we received a letter from Digna, saying she had been to church one Sunday evening with an old school friend, to a faith-healing service conducted by young Americans. One of them, coming down the aisle, looked straight at Digna and asked, 'Are you alright? Would you like me to pray for you?'

'Tell him how you feel,' her friend said.

Taken aback by his abruptness, but feeling she had nothing to lose, Digna proceeded to explain to him her fear of God, of what he might ask of her and of not being able to follow it through. The young man crouched down in front of her and took hold of her hands. He talked and prayed for 15 minutes about how much God loved her, that he loved her so much that his Son had died for her, that if he asked her to do anything to help others it would also help her, and if he asked her to give up something he would replace it with something much, much better.

'As he prayed,' Digna reported, 'I started to cry very loudly, and then I began to shiver uncontrollably, but of warmth not of cold.'

The young American explained, 'When you cried you were letting go of all your fears and anxieties about God, and the warmth was God's love replacing all the gaps.'

Digna wrote all this in the letter, and at the end she said, 'I really feel a different person.' And you can imagine our gratitude at this miracle of God while we were 3,000 miles away.

When we came home, shortly after, she really was a different young woman. Also, unknown to us, she had decided to quit the flat she had been sharing with the other girl and to come home again. Disillusioned with the hairdressing, she took up a secretarial training, at which she did very well indeed.

A friend invited her to an MRA youth camp in Norway, where she met her future husband, and now she is married to Peter Nelson of Sweden, who works in the Volvo car company in Gothenburg. In the same year Edith Anne married an American, John Gardner. They live in Iowa City, where they both are studying, and she is also able to pursue her acting career.

It was hard to see our girls leave home, this time for good – except for visits of course – but we felt very happy with their choice of husbands and we keep in touch and visit as often as possible. To our great joy we became grandparents recently. Digna and Peter had a little boy, and when I told Digna that Tim was the most beautiful baby to hit the deck this century she retorted, 'What about me?'

Annejet comes from a family of seven children. Her parents have been married for 62 years and are convinced they would never have stayed together if they had not learnt early in their married life to listen to the voice of truth inside, to say sorry when necessary, and start again from a clean slate.

206

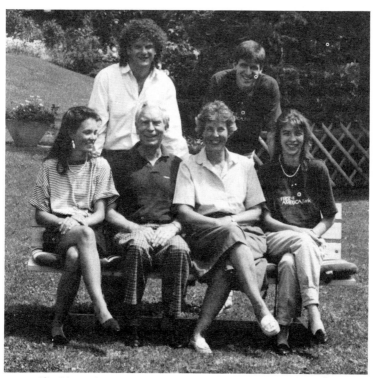

'God has given us a marvellously rich family relationship.'

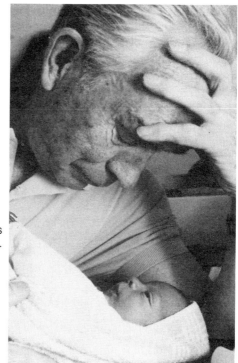

With Digna and Peter's
son Tim.

Some years ago Annejet and I were invited to meet a professional man and his wife at dinner one evening, neighbours of our hosts. The slamming of doors and shouting that came from the next-door apartment had led our hosts to try and help. Some time later the neighbours themselves invited us to their apartment for dinner.

He is Italian and his wife is Irish. They have three children - two boys and a girl. You might, with reason, imagine the Italian and Irish temperaments to be an explosive chemical mix.

A few days after our dinner the Italian called me on the phone to invite me to a Chinese restaurant for a meal. We talked for four hours. His problem, as he saw it, was that the last time his wife had gone home to Ireland she had stayed away three months. She was planning another trip the following week.

His question was, should he take out a court injunction to prevent her taking the children with her?

I replied that only he could decide, but if he was really honest about his life, inspiration might come as to what was the right course of action.

He said he would like to make the experiment. We were silent for a few minutes. Then he said, 'I have an idea. You see this suit I'm wearing, and you know the silver in my home? I got it all very cheap, because it is stolen property. I didn't steal it myself, of course, I just bought it from the people who did.

'You raise a difficult question when you say that if you have done something wrong you must find a way to put it right. I have no idea from whom the stuff was stolen, so how can I put it right?'

This again resulted in a few moments of thought. The only idea I had was to suggest to my Italian friend that he talk to his priest at the Cathedral.

Shortly after this evening, that is exactly what he did. The priest's response was, 'I'll tell you what to do. You bring a bag to me with everything "hot" you have bought, and I will take it to the police for you.'

So my friend did – three bags full. The only item he didn't bring was a fur coat which he had given to his wife. She objected to his taking it back, saying, 'I didn't buy it. I didn't steal it. It is not going to the police!'

We agreed that it was something for his wife to decide, but that he should go ahead with what he felt to be right about the rest of the items.

The fur coat story finished well. When his wife returned from Dublin, my Italian friend said he wanted her measured for her Christmas present – a new coat.

She replied, 'Oh good – I need one! While I was in Dublin I met a woman who needed that fur coat more than I did, so I gave it to her!'

One day I met my friend on his business premises. He told me he had had another idea. 'Some business men here on Oxford Street keep one set of accounts, some keep two – one for themselves and one for the Inland Revenue. I keep three – an extra set for my staff! I am going to see the Tax people to get my accounts straightened out and pay them what I owe.'

July 2nd, 1979 was an important day for Annejet and myself. It was the press launching of Annejet's first book, *Listen to the Children*. For some years she had been working closely with people concerned about the family life of the country, and wanting to help families find a faith at the heart of the home. A book seemed to be a useful and constructive contribution, so she decided to make a collection of stories from people in different countries about their experiences of raising children, and how they tackled problems from temper-tantrums in small children to drug-taking in teenagers.

Annejet's strong conviction, which I whole-heartedly share, is that sound family life is the foundation stone for our society. It is what started her collecting stories for a second book, *Listen for a Change – making marriage work*. 'Why change partners,' she says, 'when both partners can change!'

With this book she wanted to give hope that people can change, marriages can be remade, and can be an endless adventure rather than the end of adventure.

We have had a lot of fun promoting the books, travelling widely together in Europe and North America, and also Brazil, ever since they were first published. I guess it has been a salutary experience for me to become known as 'Mrs Campbell's husband'.

We were invited to Quito, Ecuador to visit friends we had not seen for 28 years. We had kept in touch by letter and exchanged Christmas cards.

We were privileged to take part in a conference in Guatemala, initiated by the only Indian woman Member of Parliament there. We went together with Regena Crowchild, Arnold's widow. The story of how her husband stopped drinking and how their marriage was saved made a great impact on those who heard it. More than 60% of the population there are Indian.

In Guatemala I met an Indian doctor who told me how difficult it was to establish health centres in the villages. Later I was able to get five used microscopes for him from my old medical school in Alberta.

Once Annejet and I were on the radio in Montréal from midnight to 3 am, talking about her books and answering questions. As the coffee machine had broken down it was quite hard work!

At a dinner party in Calgary I told a woman, 'You should get my wife's book, it tells you how to change your husband.'

'Oh', she replied, 'I'll take two!'

Her books were also on display, along with other MRA titles, at the International Book Fair in Moscow in 1989. Annejet and I jumped at this matchless chance to visit the Soviet Union, and booked ourselves a package tour to Leningrad (as it then still was) and Moscow.

What an experience. We had to pinch ourselves to believe that we were really there. The beauty of old St. Petersburg is breath-taking, and a stark contrast to the dreary modern buildings and grey lives of the people of those years. So much has changed since then, and is changing every day.

At the Book Fair we met publishers from Moscow and Lithuania who have since decided to print both Annejet's books in Russian and Lithuanian.

The world cannot exist half-slave and half-free, nor can it exist half-poor and half-prosperous. We must find a way to share the wealth and feed the hungry. Otherwise greedy men and greedy groups will invoke more and more controls, and condition millions to welcome a dictatorship.

Materialism robs men and nations of the fruits of liberty, and eventually of liberty itself. Faith is the soil of liberty. Obedience to God is the seed of liberty.

We must match our love of liberty with a love for people, and secure our freedom with the discipline of our lives, the unselfishness and honesty of our motives and our conduct, and the purity of our commitment to make the voice of God the will of the people.

One thing above all others Annejet and I have learned is that, in spite of the natural parental instinct to smooth the way for one's children, that is not the way to help them find a faith.

A robust faith is something you get by knowing what to do when it is tough, not just when it is easy. If a son or daughter can acquire the habit of listening to the Almighty then they can always get a sense of direction. No matter how difficult things may seem at that moment, there is always a way to find out what to do next.

I will be 80 soon. My life has turned out totally different from the one I had planned for myself – to be a clinical expert at some prestigious University. When I made that difficult decision to resign from the Henry Ford Hospital in 1942, little did I expect the years of tremendous adventure and richness that followed.

It has been beyond anything I deserved or anticipated. To me the most satisfying thing in life is to see the spirit of God at work in the life of another person, and to see that person develop into a potential leader for his or her nation.

I love Canada. I am proud to be a Canadian. I have faith in the future of our magnificent country.

PHOTO ACKNOWLEDGMENTS

All pictures are personal photographs belonging to the Campbell family with the exception of the following:

p29: My ambition; Guy Woolford   p47: Buchman and Paul; MRA Archive
p47: Friendship; Arthur Strong   p61: With Peter Howard; David Channer
p61: New Zealand; MRA Archive   p73: Wedding photo; Arthur Strong
p83: Mackinac Island, Walking Buffalo; MRA Archive
p101: Forgotten Factor; Arthur Strong   p101: Ladder; Harold White
p127: Edith Anne with Digna; Arthur Strong   p.127 Asia Plateau school; MRA Archive
p149: T Elwood and C Hunte; Jean Normandiu   p149: Drew Webster, J Pellerin; Richard Weeks
p163: Irish with Trois Rivieres Mayor; Roland Lemire
p163: Chief John Snow/Peace pipe and p169: Arnold Crowchild; Richard Weeks
p169: Chiefs at Calgary Airport and p181: Campfire; Lars Rengfelt
p181: Nelson Small Legs Jnr; Richard Weeks   p191: Teepees; Lars Rengfelt
p191: Pow-wow; Richard Weeks
Back cover; Susan Faber